THE CLINICAL LABORATORY MANUAL SERIES:

Immunology

Juanita A. Smith

THE CLINICAL LABORATORY MANUAL SERIES:

Immunology

Juanita A. Smith

Delmar Publishers™

I Ⓣ P An International Thomson Publishing Company

Albany • Bonn • Boston • Cincinnati • Detroit • London • Madrid • Melbourne
Mexico City • New York • Pacific Grove • Paris • San Francisco • Singapore • Tokyo
Toronto • Washington

NOTICE TO THE READER

Delmar Staff

Administrative Editor: Marion Waldman   Production Coordinator: John Mickelbank
Project Editor: Megan A. Terry

COPYRIGHT © 1995
By Delmar Publishers
a division of International Thomson Publishing Inc.
The ITP logo is a trademark under license
Printed in the United States of America

For more information, contact:

Delmar Publishers
3 Columbia Circle, Box 15015
Albany, New York 12212-5015

International Thomson Publishing Europe
Berkshire House 168-173
High Holborn
London WC1V 7AA
England

Thomas Nelson Australia
102 Dodds Street
South Melbourne, 3205
Victoria, Australia

Nelson Canada
1120 Birchmount Road
Scarborough, Ontario
Canada M1K 5G4

International Thomson Editores
Campos Eliseos 385, Piso 7
Col Polanco
11560 Mexico D F Mexico

International Thomson Publishing GmbH
Königswinterer Strasse 418
53227 Bonn
Germany

International Thomson Publishing Asia
221 Henderson Road
#05-10 Henderson Building
Singapore 0315

International Thomson Publishing Japan
Hirakawacho Kyowa Building, 3F
2-2-1 Hirakawacho
Chiyoda-ku, Tokyo 102
Japan

1 2 3 4 5 6 7 8 9 10   xxx   01 00 99 98 97 96 95

Library of Congress Cataloging-in-Publication Data
Smith, Juanita A.
    Immunology / Juanita A. Smith.
      p.   cm. — (The clinical laboratory manual series)
    Includes bibliographical references and index.
    ISBN 0-8273-5637-4
    1. Immunodiagnosis—Laboratory manuals.   2. Immunology—Laboratory manuals.   I. Title.   II. Series.
    (DNLM: 1. Immunologic Tests—laboratory manuals.   2. Immunologic Techniques.   3. Serodiagnosis—laboratory manuals.   QW 525 S653i 1995]
RB46.5.S65 1995
616.07′56—dc20
DNLM/DLC
for Library of Congress
                94-41922
                CIP

ACKNOWLEDGMENTS

I wish to thank all of the people who have encouraged the writing of this document, including Marion Waldman, editor, Health Sciences, who answered a multitude of questions; Jacquelyn Marshall, Medical Laboratory Manual Series editor, who gave encouragement and boosted my confidence when it was needed.

The manuscript reviewers:
Sally McLaughlin Baeur
Hudson Valley Community College
Troy, New York

Sharon Bramson
The College of Staten Island
Staten Island, New York

Susan Strasinger
Northern Virginia Community College
Annandale, Virginia

Also, I thank my daughters. Ardis did the drawings and provided me with assistance on the computer. Denise was my proofreader and gave me constant encouragement.

CONTENTS

■ **Contents**

Contents ▪

LIST OF LABORATORY EXERCISES

PREFACE

This laboratory manual is written for the medical laboratory technician student. The manual is also an excellent review for medical technicians or technologists who need a refresher in immunology. This manual was written to provide a hands-on learning guide for students with a limited science background. Included are class activities, test procedures, and case studies. Questions at the end of each chapter reinforce material previously learned.

Many of the textbooks currently available for medical laboratory technician students are excellent, but there is too much information to wade through. It is our hope that this manual presents vital information to the medical laboratory technician and creates excitement about the field of immunology. This manual may be used as a stand alone in the laboratory environment or as a study aid to augment any immunology textbook.

Following are some of the highlights of each unit.

Unit 1 reviews the type of antigens and the introduction of the antigens into the human body. The response of the body to antigens is also covered.

Unit 2 covers the important safety precautions that must be taken while one is working in a laboratory, the need for quality assurance in regard to each serological test procedure, and the importance of keeping accurate records.

Unit 3 reviews syphilis serology and the results of untreated syphilis and covers nontreponemal and treponemal test procedures.

Unit 4 discusses the common viral diseases encountered in the serology testing area. Included are hepatitis, acquired immunodeficiency syndrome, and cytomegalovirus.

Unit 5 covers common febrile diseases and test procedures for the diseases. The unit discusses the response of C-reactive protein to inflammation. Also included is serological test procedures for the exoenzymes produced in the human body to streptococcal infections.

Unit 6 is devoted to the two most common autoimmune diseases, systematic lupus erythematosus and rheumatoid arthritis.

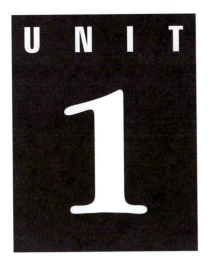

Immunology Overview

LEARNING OBJECTIVES

After studying this unit, the student should know the following objectives:

- Discuss types of antigen response.

- Name and discuss types of immunity.

- State characteristics of an antigen.

- Name chemical properties of an antigen.

- Give types of antigen reactions.

- Name five classes of immunoglobulins.

- Discuss a mechanism for termination of antibody production.

- Discuss cells of the immune system.

- Give stages of the complement pathway.

- Discuss types of reactions that take place in serology procedures.

GLOSSARY

Anamnestic response: Rapid reappearance of antibody following exposure to an antigen to which the person has already developed a response.

Angstrom unit: Measurement of length, 1/10,000 of a micron (μ).

Antibody: Immunoglobulin (protein) produced in response to antigen stimulation (immunoglobulin).

Antigen: Protein foreign to the body of the host-creating antibody response in the immunocompetent individual.

Autoimmune: Abnormal production of antibody against self; self acts as the antigen.

B cell: Lymphocyte; white blood cells of the immune system producing antibody (humoral response).

Carrier portion: Soluble portion of the antigen with determinants recognized by T lymphocytes.

CD markers: Clusters of differentiation on T lymphocytes and other types of lymphocytes.

Complement: Protein found in normal serum that aids in phagocytosis and in antigen-antibody reactions.

Dalton: An arbitrary unit of mass equal to $\frac{1}{12}$ the mass of carbon 12.

Determinate portion: Portion of an antigen that determines specificity with an antibody.

Exudate: Fluid produced in response to inflammation containing white blood cells.

Fibrinogen: Protein found in plasma that aids in clot formation.

Hapten(e): Small protein capable of binding with carbohydrate-lipid complexes to produce antibody.

Hemolysis: Destruction of a red blood cell with loss of hemoglobin.

Immunity: State in which the body is resistant to disease.

Immunocompetent: Capability to produce antibody against a foreign protein.

Immunocompromised: Reduced or absent capability to produce antibody against a foreign protein.

Immunoglobulin: Antibodies produced by the body.

Immunology: Science dealing with resistance to disease-producing organisms.

In vitro: Outside of the body (e.g., in a test tube).

In vivo: Inside of the body (e.g., in life).

Leukocyte: White blood cell (WBC).

Lymphocyte: Type of white blood cell.

Lysozyme: Enzyme present in tears and saliva secreted by macrophages.

Macrophage: Mononuclear cell (white blood cells) that phagocytizes foreign material.

Mast cell: Cell found in tissue that produces and stores histamine and other mediators.

Natural killer (NK) cell: Lymphocyte, neither T nor B.

Neonate: Newborn.

Neutrophil: Type of white blood cell.

Normal flora: Microorganisms normally present in or on the body.

Phagocytosis: Engulfment and destruction of foreign particles.

Plasma: Liquid portion of the blood after it has been anticoagulated.

Plasma cells: Cells formed when B cells (lymphocytes) are stimulated to replicate by contact with antigen.

Serology: Study of serum.

Serum: Liquid portion remaining after the blood has clotted.

T cell: Lymphocyte responsible for cellular immune response.

Transudate: A fluid that passes through membranes (e.g., capillary walls).

INTRODUCTION

Immunology is the science that deals with the body's ability to react to foreign substances **(antigens)** and its resistance to disease-producing organisms. **Serology** is the study of serum for **antibody** response to exposed microorganisms, allergy-producing substances, **autoimmune** antigens, and parasites.

The immune phenomenon was first recognized in association with smallpox. Louis Jenner's work with smallpox gave us the term "vaccine." This term is still used today for injected preparations that stimulate tissues to produce immunity to a specific disease. The agents administered are **antigens** or foreign proteins. The substances produced in response to the antigen are **antibodies**.

IMMUNITY

The function of the immune system is to recognize self from non-self and to defend the body from non-self. In the **immunocompetent** systems, the body is capable of discerning self from non-self. In the immunosuppressed individual, the body is incapable of the recognition of self from non-self. Substances that are non-self are microorganisms, bacteria, and viruses. In the immunosuppressed system, the body will slowly form or will not form an antibody to the foreign particles. For example, people who are infected with the acquired immune deficiency syndrome (AIDS) virus are immunosuppressed as the disease progresses, and the body will not form antibodies to foreign antigens. In the immunocompetent system, antibody will be produced in reaction to the foreign protein particles.

The human body has many barriers to prevent invasion by foreign particles. The main barrier is intact skin. Another barrier, the mucosal membrane, contains IgA antibodies and **lysozymes** and is considered a chemical means of protection. Lysozymes (enzymes) are also present in saliva and tears, as well as in **neutrophils** and **macrophages**. The acidity level of the stomach fluids destroys microorganisms, as does the **normal flora** in the upper portion of the intestinal tract. Normal flora consists of microorganisms present in and on the body to give the body protection from disease processes.

E X E R C I S E **1** **VACCINES**

Divide the class into groups and have a discussion on the administration of vaccines and the results received from the injections.

1. Discuss different vaccines for diseases.
2. Discuss how the vaccine protects the body from diseases.
3. Discuss immunizations given to protect the health care worker.

E X E R C I S E   **2**   **IMMUNE SYSTEM**

Divide the class into groups and discuss the following:

1. How the immunocompetent system protects the body.
2. How the immunosuppressed system fails to protect the body.
3. What can be done to improve the immune system.

Table 1.1. Components of the Immune System that Respond Readily to Bodily Invasion of Foreign Antigens

Cellular	**Humoral**
Macrophages	Antibodies
Neutrophils	Complement
B lymphocytes	Interferon
T lymphocytes	Lysozyme
Plasma cells	

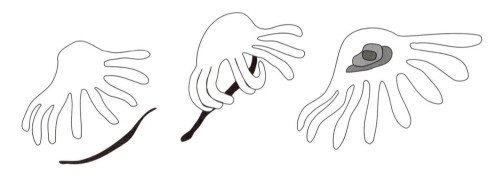

fig. 1.1. Macrophage attacking bacteria

TYPES OF IMMUNE RESPONSES

Two types of responses are produced by the host in response to antigen. The first response is cellular response (Table 1.1). This response is caused by the penetration of a foreign agent that causes inflammation. Inflammation is a condition that causes tissues to become swollen with redness, heat, and pain. Blood vessels dilate to let a greater volume of blood flow to the injury. Acute inflammation consists of the formation of an **exudate**, which contains fluid, cells, and antibacterial substances. **Fibrinogen** (a protein in **serum** or **plasma**) is converted to fibrin to form a clot, which aids in connecting tissue and is a barrier against bacteria. Fibrin, macrophages, neutrophils, and **mast cells** aid in **phagocytosis**.

Phagocytosis is the engulfment of foreign particles, including microorganisms, by a variety of cells in the body. White blood cells (leukocytes) are the most well known of the cells that phagocytize foreign particles. The cellular response to inflammation begins when white blood cells enter the injury site (Figure 1.1). They adhere to the vessel wall and push pseudopodia (false feet) between endothelial cells (cells lining vessels) and emerge on the external surface.

5

The first cells to appear in cellular exudate are the neutrophils (Figure 1.2). The second cells to appear are the monocytes (known as macrophages). Lymphocytes are also present in the exudate. In viral penetration, lymphocytes will be the predominant cells.

The second response is humoral response. Humoral response is the response of the host to produce antibody to the invading organism. The humoral components of the immune system are **complement** (a protein), lysozyme (an enzyme), and interferon (an antiviral substance).

Neutrophil 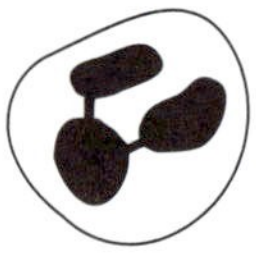	Cell with three to five lobes; cytoplasm stains pink-lavender.
Lymphocyte 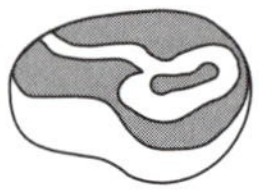	Cell with round or oval nucleus; cytoplasm stains blue.
Monocyte 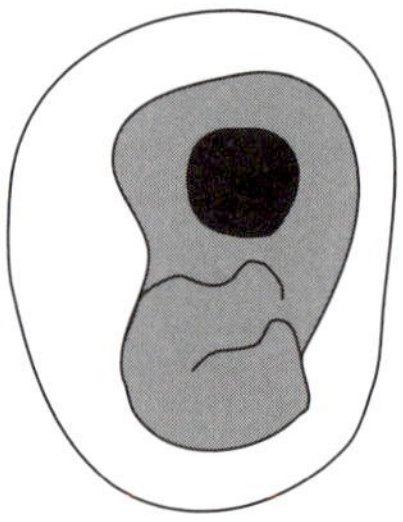	Large white blood cell with nucleus shaped like a lima bean; cytoplasm stains gray-blue.
Eosinophil 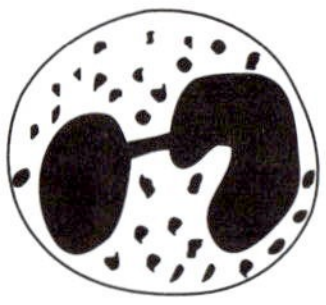	Cell with two nuclei and large granules; cytoplasm contains large stained red/orange granules.
Basophil 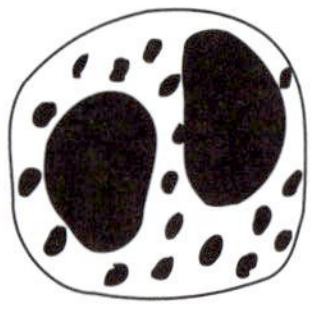	Cell with large granules; the cytoplasm stains dark purple.

fig. 1.2. White blood cells

TYPES OF IMMUNITY

Immunity can be classified under two broad terms: naturally acquired and artificially acquired. Naturally acquired immunity is present at birth. The antibody detected in serum of the **neonate** has been passively transferred from the maternal circulation. This type of immunity has a short life span, often referred to as passive acquired immunity.

Other types of naturally acquired immunity result from contact with foreign proteins by the host with no obvious disease process involved, but the host can have a subclinical disease process. Penetration of foreign substances into the body that cause disease with production of antibody (also classified under naturally acquired immunity) is often referred to as active acquired immunity. The antibody produced is usually specific for the antigen that caused its production.

Some antigen-antibody reactions confer lifetime immunity to the disease-producing organisms. Chicken pox is an example of a disease that produces lifetime immunity to future exposure; in other words, once you have had chicken pox, you can never get it again. An example of a disease that does not confer lifetime immunity is syphilis. Syphilis can be contracted again and again with each exposure.

Artificial immunity is stimulated by the introduction of artificial antigens or antibodies into the individual. This procedure requires the production of antibodies in an individual or an animal. These antibodies are then purified and prepared into solutions, which are then injected into another individual, protecting the injected individual from the disease. The material injected is called a vaccine. The injection of a vaccine does not confer lifetime immunity. The injections must be given periodically to maintain an antibody titer. An antibody titer is the amount of antibody present in the serum to protect the injected individual from the disease. For a quick overview of which vaccines are or are not available for common diseases, see Table 1.2.

Certain species are resistant to certain diseases. For example, humans do not acquire canine parvovirus, and canines do not acquire rubella. The resistance to some diseases appears to be genetically controlled. For example, individuals who do not inherit Duffy antigens appear to be resistant to certain strains of malaria. Duffy antigens are genetic material inherited on the red blood cell.

Some humans are carriers of disease-producing organisms. These individuals, such as Typhoid Mary, do not have active symptoms of the disease but are capable of transferring the disease-producing organism to others. She carried the typhoid organism (*Salmonella*) but never became ill herself. In her work as a domestic, she passed the typhoid organism on to her employers and their families.

To enter some health care schools in the United States, it is mandatory for the prospective student to have MMR immunizations. It is highly recommended that the student also be immunized against hepatitis B.

Table 1.2. Vaccine Availability

Vaccines available	No vaccines available
Diptheria, pertussis, and tetanus (DPT)	Malaria
Measles, mumps, and rubella (MMR)	Infectious mononucleosis
Hepatitis B	Hepatitis A

EXERCISE   **3**   **IMMUNITY DISCUSSION**

Have a class discussion about diseases causing short-term immunity and lifetime immunity.

1. Name organisms that will produce short-term immunity and the diseases they produce.
2. Discuss how the disease affects the body.
3. Name organisms that will produce lifetime immunity and the diseases they produce.
4. Discuss how the disease affects the body.

EXERCISE   **4**   **DISEASE TRANSMISSION**

Have a class discussion on different ways diseases are transmitted.

1. Nurse working in newborn nursery who has a *Staphylococcus* infection in her nose.
2. Children ill with measles in a day-care center.
3. Individuals with AIDS.

Individuals of the same species demonstrate differences in susceptibility and nonsusceptibility. These differences are seen in different races, age groups, and genders. The presence or absence of certain hormones can also influence susceptibility. For example, women become more susceptible to cancers when their estrogen production is reduced or altered. As people age, the immune system does not work as well. That is why older people are more susceptible to influenza or other illnesses. Some races are immune to certain disease processes due to their genetic inheritance; for example, the absence of Duffy antigens makes one resistant to malaria. Duffy antigens are inherited antigens on the surface of the red blood cell.

Antigens are protein agents that enter the body and cause a response to the agent. This response is usually in the form of an antibody. Examples of antigens are microorganisms, toxins, pollens, food substances, or red blood cells.

To be classified as an antigen, the protein must have certain characteristics. The protein must (1) gain entry into the body, (2) be foreign to the body, (3) have a high molecular weight (i.e., 10,000 **daltons** or greater), and (4) have a high order of specificity. Specificity is defined as the ability of a particular antibody to bind with one antigen with complimentary determinants. In addition, the antigen must be capable of reacting in a demonstrable way with the antibody produced by that specific antigen.

The chemical properties of an antigen consist of lipoproteins, carbohydrate-protein complexes, and polysaccharides. Antigens are composed of two parts: a **carrier portion**, which is a soluble carrier of the antigen into the host; and a **determinate portion**, which gives the antigen its specificity as a foreign protein to the host for the production of antibody.

Some proteins do not have all of the characteristics necessary to be classified as an antigen. If the protein is small, it must combine with other components to be antigenic. An example of this is the **hapten(e)**, which can consist of carbohydrates (sugars), proteins, amino acids, or inorganic radicals. When the carrier portion and a hapten(e) combine, there will be production of a specific antibody for the protein.

Antigens are given different classifications by their reaction in testing procedures. Complete antigens are those antigens that stimulate antibody formation and will react in a visible manner, demonstrating activity by agglutination (clumping of cells) or lysis (destruction of cells). Soluble antigens are those in which the **in vitro** reaction (in a tube) is demonstrated by complement fixation or precipitation (formation of particles in a solution).

In autoimmune diseases, the immune system does not distinguish self from non-self antigens and will produce antibody against self. Table 1.3 lists several common autoimmune diseases.

Antibodies are proteins produced in response to an antigen. These proteins are known as globulins. The fractions (parts) of globulins are designated as alpha (α), beta (β), and gamma (γ). Antibodies are found in the serum or plasma fraction of the blood. Other terms for antibody are **immune globulin** or **immunoglobulin**. This term is used because these globulins take part in the immune response. Some immunoglobulins are produced by B lymphocytes that have changed their characteristics and have turned into plasma cells.

There are five main classes of immunoglobulins identified in humans: IgG, IgM, IgA, IgD, and IgE. These globulins have basic structural characteristics but vary in size and weight (Table 1.4). The antibodies have two heavy (hc) and two light peptide chains (lc) linked by disulfide bonds at the "hinge" area of the structure. Each structure has a Fab and Fc part. The Fab portion is capable of binding antigen. The Fc portion is responsible for adherence of the antibody to the surface of the monocyte in cell-mediated responses. The hinge portion of the antibody activates the complement pathway.

Table 1.3. Types of Autoimmune Diseases

Rheumatoid arthritis
Systemic lupus erythematosus
Diabetes mellitus
Hemolytic anemia

Table 1.4. Size and Structure of Immunoglobulins

	IgM	IgA	IgG	IgD	IgE
MW daltons	900,000	180,000–500,000	150,000	180,000	200,000
Sediment coefficient	19 S	7–15 S	6–7 S	7 S	8 S
Size in **Angstrom** units	1,000	250	250	250	250

CLASSES OF IMMUNOGLOBULINS

Immunoglobulin G (IgG) is the most abundant immunoglobulin found in the serum and is composed of two light and two heavy chains and has two binding sites. IgG also contains subunits (IgG1, IgG2, IgG3, and IgG4). It has the capacity to fix subunits of complement and the capacity to agglutinate cells. It reacts against microorganisms and toxins in extracellular fluids. It is produced later in the immune response and has a long life.

Immunoglobulin M (IgM) is made up of five structural units formed in a circle. The five units are linked together by a chain (J chain). The immunoglobulin M has 10 binding sites (Figure 1.3). It has the capacity for strong agglutination and complement fixation. It is produced early in the immune response but stops production within a few weeks.

Immunoglobulin A (IgA) has two distinct forms. Some IgA is found in the serum and some in secretions. Ninety percent of serum IgA has two antigen or binding sites. The other 10% exists with four or six binding sites. Secretory IgA is found in saliva, tears, and mucous membranes. It plays an important role in the first line of defense of the body against invading microorganisms and other foreign macromolecules.

Immunoglobulin D (IgD) is composed of two light chains and two heavy chains. It has two binding sites. Very little is known about the function of IgD. It is found at times on the surface of B lymphocytes.

Immunoglobulin E (IgE) is associated with allergic reactions. It is often found in elevated quantities in patients with parasitic infections. In allergic reactions IgE will be elevated from the more severe anaphylactic reactions to milder forms of allergies.

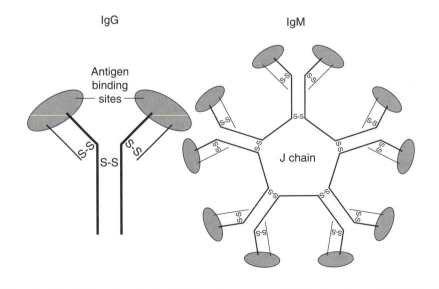

fig. 1.3. IgG and IgM

CASE STUDY ■ **ALLERGIC REACTIONS**

A patient has entered the hospital emergency room with multiple bee stings. The patient is having trouble breathing. What is causing the breathing difficulty?

1. Discuss the reaction to bee stings in different people. Include allergic and immune responses.
2. What is the reaction that causes swelling?
3. Discuss what immunoglobulin will be increased with bee stings.

IMMUNE RESPONSE

When an antigen enters the body, the immune system will start antibody production. The antibody will usually appear five to seven days after antigen exposure. The first class of antibody to appear is IgM. The IgM antibody will diminish, and the body will begin to produce an IgG form of the antibody that is a longer-lasting antibody. The IgG antibody will diminish in time and may become undetectable in the serum or plasma. This response is called the primary response.

If the body is challenged with an antigen again, the antibody to the antigen will appear in the circulatory system within 24 to 48 hours. This quick response is called a secondary response, **anamnestic response**, or recall phenomenon.

The antibody produced in this response is IgG, and it will be produced in large quantities. The IgG antibody will have a higher binding constant and will remain in the system for a longer time than the IgM antibody produced in the primary response. Ultimately this antibody may also become undetectable. The antigen dosage can be much smaller for the secondary response than the antigen dosage that started the primary response. As little as 0.1 ml of antigen is capable of initiating the anamnestic response.

CELLS OF THE IMMUNE SYSTEM

Several cells of the immune system aid in the immune response in the immunocompetent individual. The cells involved are macrophages, monocytes, and cells with presenting antigens. Also included in this grouping are B cells and T cells (lymphocytes) (Figure 1.4).

The presenting antigen cells are monocytes, macrophages, and other cells in the body that are macrophages, including microglial cells and Kupffer's cells. The latter two cell types are responsible for the release of interleukin I.

T cells are produced in the bone marrow and migrate to the thymus, where they mature and then migrate to the bloodstream. T cells have clusters of differentiation (CD). The **CD markers** on T cells give the cells classification. The T cells of greatest concern in **immunocompromised** individuals are CD T4 and CD T8 cells. The CD T4 cells are helper cells, and CD T8 cells have two designa-

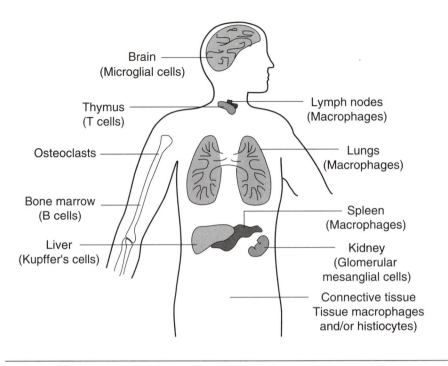

fig. 1.4. Cells of the immune system

tions: T suppressor cells and cytotoxic T cells. The T cells are responsible for recognizing foreign proteins entering the body.

B cells are produced in the bone marrow and migrate to the circulatory system. These cells undergo changes to become **plasma cells**, which produce immunoglobulins (antibodies) to a foreign protein. The immature B cell does not change into a mature cell until it has been exposed to an antigen. It then will produce immunoglobulin that is specific for the invading antigen.

Other cells are K cells (null cells). These cells are neither T cells nor B cells. They are not macrophages. K cells cannot kill target cells unless a specific antibody is present.

Natural killer (NK) cells are **lymphocytes** that do not have B- or T-lymphocyte receptors and are not phagocytic. They possess cytotoxic characteristics that will kill organisms such as viruses.

REGULATION OF THE IMMUNE RESPONSE

Four mechanisms regulate the amount of antibody produced and terminate antibody production.

In the first mechanism, plasma cells survive only a few days, and unless new plasma cells evolve, antibody production ceases.

In the second mechanism, an antibody produced in an immune response coats the macrophage-bound antigen so it no longer stimulates antibody production.

In the third mechanism, suppressor T cells (Ts) are activated, which causes them to inhibit stimulation of other lymphocytes.

Finally, in the fourth mechanism, the antigen that initiated the response is often degraded or eliminated from the body.

E X E R C I S E | 5 | AIDS PATIENT CELL COUNT

1. Discuss the action of B and T cells in an AIDS patient.
2. Discuss why it is necessary for the AIDS patient to have repeated T-cell lymphocyte counts.
3. Discuss what happens when the T-cell count is very low in the AIDS patient.

THE COMPLEMENT SYSTEM

Complement is the name of a group of 11 different serum proteins. These serum proteins are known as C_1 (which has three components q, r, and s), C_2, C_3, C_4, C_5, C_6, C_7, C_8, and C_9. Complement is composed of globulins, which, as mentioned earlier, play an important part in antigen-antibody reactions. Complement activation has two pathways: classical and alternative.

The complement cascade can be activated by IgM, IgG1, IgG2, and IgG3 antibodies.

Complement is found in fresh serum and will be inactivated or denatured by heating the serum to 56°C. For the complement cascade to progress from C_1 to C_9, calcium and magnesium must be present.

For the classical pathway to be activated, C_1q must be fixed to the cell site. When C_1q is fixed to the cell, a component of C_1 will be formed that consists of C_1q, C_1r, and C_1s. Calcium must be present at this point for the C_1 complex to be held together. Once C_1 is attached to the cell, C_4 attaches to the cell. Then, C_2 is the next component of complement to attach to the cell. Magnesium must be present at this phase. The process will continue from this point on in a logical manner, with the attachment of C_3, C_5, C_6, C_7, C_8, and C_9 (Figure 1.5).

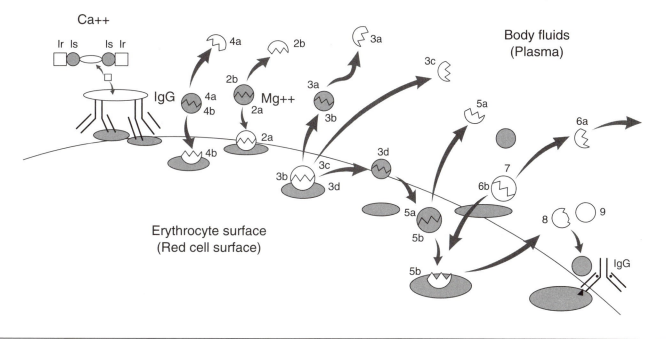

fig. 1.5. Complement fixation: the classical pathway

When all of the components of complement have attached to the cell, a lesion will be formed in the red blood cell membrane, and hemoglobin will be released, resulting in hemolysis of the cell.

The alternative pathway does not require the activation of C_1, C_4, or C_2. The pathway begins with activation of C_3 and proceeds through the pathway to C_9 and cell destruction. Polysaccharides (sugars), enzymes, or antigen-antibody complexes will activate the alternative pathway.

TYPES OF ANTIGENS

Laboratory test procedures in immunology demonstrate **hemolysis**, agglutination, or complement fixation. These reactions are the result of different types of antigen-antibody reactions. See Table 1.5.

TEST PROCEDURE REACTIONS

The following reactions are those found most frequently in serological test procedures.

Agglutination reactions are those in which a cellular (red blood cell) or particulate antigen (a latex particle) is suspended in a fluid and reacted with serum to determine if an antibody is present. If a reaction takes place between the antigen in the suspension and an antibody in the serum being tested, the cells or particulate matter will settle out in clumps. An example of this type of procedure is the Monospot test for the detection of infectious mononucleosis.

Precipitation reactions are those in which a soluble antigen is reacted with serum to determine the presence of antibody. If there is a reaction, a fine flocculate will develop that can be seen visually or microscopically. Two tests that demonstrate flocculation reactions are the RPR (rapid plasma reagin) and the VDRL (Venereal Disease Research Laboratory), both of which are used to detect syphilis. These procedures will be discussed in Unit 3.

Lysis reactions occur when blood cells or bacterial cells are dissolved after reacting with their specific antibody. Lysis is the destruction or breakdown of the cell used. An example of this type of procedure is the antistreptolysin O titer.

Agglutination, precipitation, and lysis are types of visible reactions. Complement fixation is an antigen-antibody reaction (Figures 1.6A and B). This test procedure needs complement to cause the antigen-antibody reaction to occur. In these procedures, if the antigen-antibody reaction takes place, there is no visible

Table 1.5. Types of Antigens

Complete antigen	Stimulates antibody formation and reacts in a visible manner, resulting in agglutination or lysis of the test particles.
Soluble antigen	Demonstrates complement fixation or precipitation in an in vitro reaction.
Haptens [hapten(e)]	Incomplete antigens that will react with specific antibody in vitro but must attach to a larger particle to produce antibody **in vivo**; the larger particle the hapten(e) attaches to is called a carrier particle.

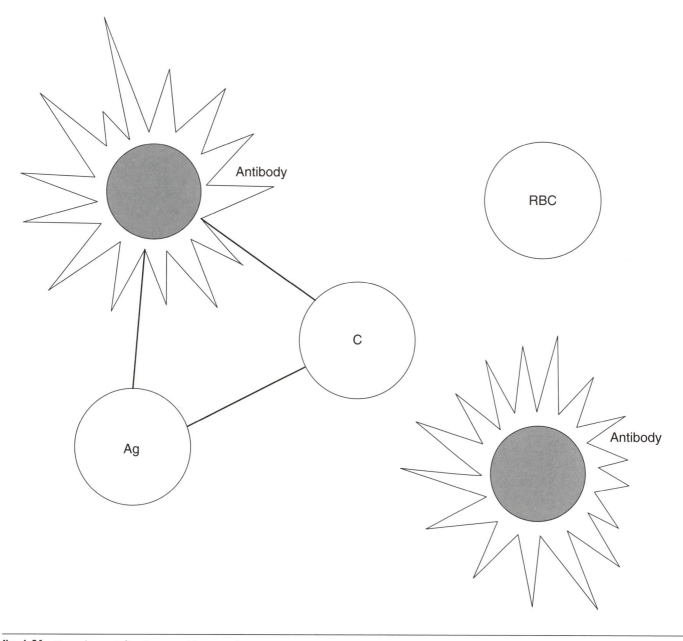

fig. 1.6A. Complement fixation: positive reactions

reaction. It is necessary to add to this reaction a second antigen-antibody indicator such as red blood cells. In this type of test, if the red blood cells *do not lyse,* it indicates that a specific antigen-antibody reaction occurred and that complement was bound and inactivated. If the *red blood cells lyse,* it indicates that the complement did not bind to the cell and a specific antigen-antibody reaction did not occur.

Passive hemagglutination (inhibition) is a method of antigen-antibody testing that does just what the name states. The reaction will be inhibited when antigen-antibody reactions occur, and there will be no agglutination of the test cells. In this procedure a positive test result has a mat of cells covering the bottom of the test well. A negative test result was a solid mass of cells in the bottom of the well. A doubling dilution of serum was prepared in a microtiter plate. Red blood cells

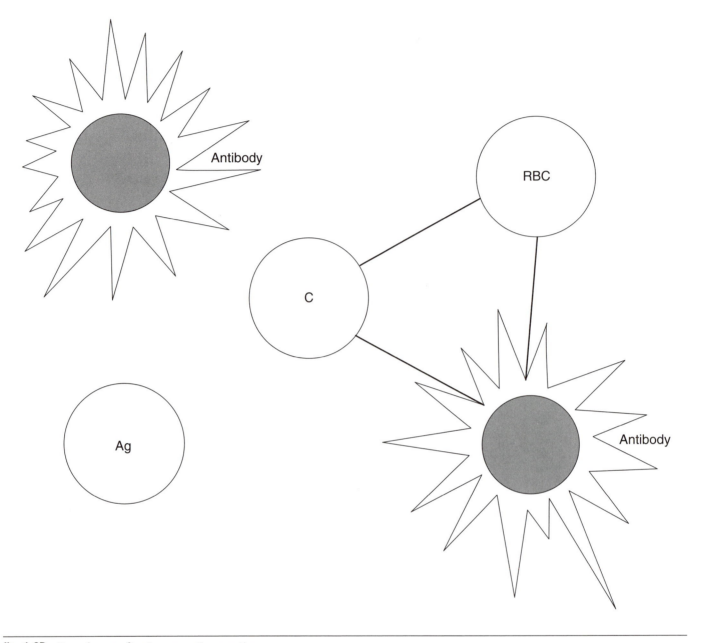

fig. 1.6B. Complement fixation: negative reactions

were then added, and the plates were placed on a flat surface for 2 hours. The test was not difficult to perform but was time consuming.

Radial immunodiffusion is used for the quantitation of serum protein, complement, and immunoglobulins. (Figure 1.7).

A protein (antigen) solution is placed in a well cut in a gel matrix that contains a known concentration of monospecific antibody. Antigen placed in the well diffuses, producing a precipitin ring.

If one is testing for C_3, a fresh serum sample must be used (less than 2 hours old). The C_3 component will break down to C_{3c} in serum as it ages.

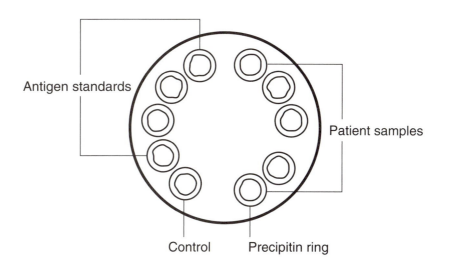

fig. 1.7. Radial immunodiffusion

EXERCISE ▪ 6 ▪ RADIAL IMMUNODIFFUSION (FIGURE 1.7)

1. Remove radial immunodiffusion plates from the refrigerator and warm to room temperature.
2. Remove plate from plastic package and remove plate cover.
3. Place 5 µl of the antigen standard solutions into wells marked for standards.
4. Place 5 µl of control solution into wells marked for control.
5. Place 5 µl of patient serum into the wells marked for patient serum.
6. Cover plate tightly and enclose in a plastic bag.
7. Place plate in a horizontal position and allow to stand for 18 hours.
8. At the end of the 18 hours, measure precipitin rings for the standards, the controls, and the patients. Calculate values for each of the patients by the formula given by the manufacturer.

Standards and controls must be performed with the patient's serum samples. The plates are incubated for 18 hours or overnight. The diameter of the precipitin ring is measured to the nearest 0.1 mm. The diameter of each precipitin ring for the standard solution is plotted on the x axis of semilog graph paper against its respective concentration, which is plotted on the y axis. The two points are connected. Values for the test samples are determined from the reference curve.

SOURCES OF ERROR

1. Distorted precipitin rings due to cuts in the agarose gel, spilling of the sample outside of the well, accidental freezing of the plate, and seepage of the sample under the gel to the bottom of the plate.

17

2. Elliptical rings due to overfilling of the well, placement of the plate on an uneven surface, drying of the agarose gel, or lids not closed correctly.
3. Double or triple rings due to filling the well twice.

OUCHTERLONY DOUBLE DIFFUSION METHOD OF IMMUNODIFFUSION

One type of antigen-antibody reaction is performed on an agar gel plate by immunodiffusion. This type of test procedure was perfected by Ouchterlony (Figure 1.8). A plate with agar gel is prepared with small wells cut into the gel. Antigen is placed in one well and patient serum is placed into the other wells. The soluble antigen will diffuse toward the antibody in the serum, forming a precipitin line. This line is called an identity line. Various lines of identity can be formed: identity, nonidentity, and partial identity.

ELECTROPHORESIS

Electrophoresis is used to determine the type of antibodies (immunoglobulins) that are present in the serum of an individual (Figure 1.9). This test is performed using a cellulose acetate strip. The serum being tested is placed on the strip. The strip is then subjected to an electric current. The different fractions of the immunoglobulins will diffuse into bands on the cellulose acetate strip. The strip is then stained and processed through a reader, which will print out a graph of the fractionation of the protein bands.

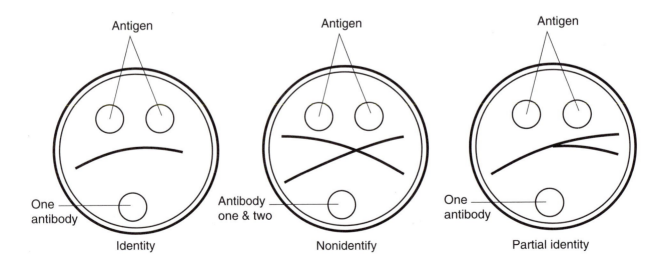

fig. 1.8. Ouchterlony double diffusion

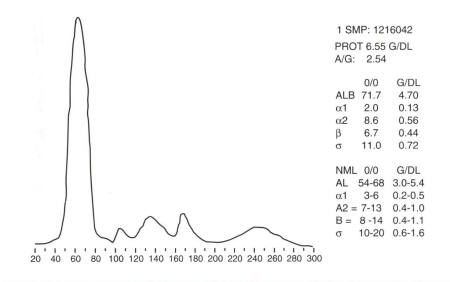

1 SMP: 1216042
PROT 6.55 G/DL
A/G: 2.54

	0/0	G/DL
ALB	71.7	4.70
α1	2.0	0.13
α2	8.6	0.56
β	6.7	0.44
σ	11.0	0.72

NML	0/0	G/DL
AL	54-68	3.0-5.4
α1	3-6	0.2-0.5
A2 =	7-13	0.4-1.0
B =	8-14	0.4-1.1
σ	10-20	0.6-1.6

fig. 1.9. Electrophoresis

IMMUNOASSAY

Immunoassay is one of the newer forms of testing in serology. These test proce-dures use enzymes in the reaction. The tests for hepatitis, rubella, and AIDS are just a few of the procedures performed by this method. These procedures are enzyme-linked immunosorbent assays, often referred to as ELISA methods (Fig-ure 1.10). The enzyme frequently used in the test procedure is a horseradish per-oxidase. The results are determined by a color change in the test solution. A printout of test results is provided in this test.

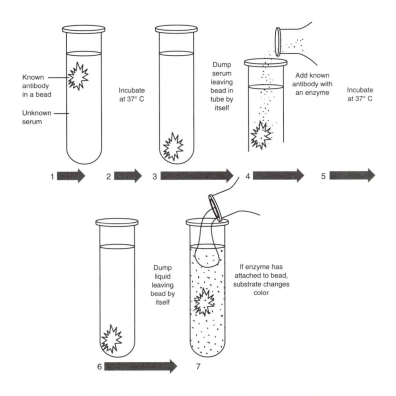

fig. 1.10. Enzyme immunosorbent reaction

AUTOMATION

There are different types of automated equipment used in serology, depending on the testing performed by the various laboratories. Some of the equipment uses fluorescence as a marker for the antigen-antibody complex, which has been stained by a fluorescent material. The FIAX fluorometer (Figure 1.11) is one type of equipment that reads fluorescence. One serological procedure performed on the FIAX is a solid-phase fluorescence immunoassay to test for antinuclear antibodies, which are found in several diseases. These diseases will be discussed in a later unit. Some of the fluorescent dyes give a green or yellow color.

Other pieces of equipment perform counts for DNA markers. This type of count is performed by flow cytometry. Flow cytometry analyzes individual cells that have been tagged with antibody. The RNA and DNA examination is determined by this method. Also the number of B and T cells can be monitored to determine the immune status of the patient. This is very important in immunocompromised patients.

In flow cell cytometry, a large number of cells will pass through an aperture in the equipment where they are exposed to light or electric current to generate a signal that is measured. Specific antibody is used to detect cell markers and will demonstrate on a scattergram the number of T_H, T_S, and B lymphocytes. Also demonstrated are NK cells and granulocytes. From the scattergram one can give a count of the cells present in the blood specimen.

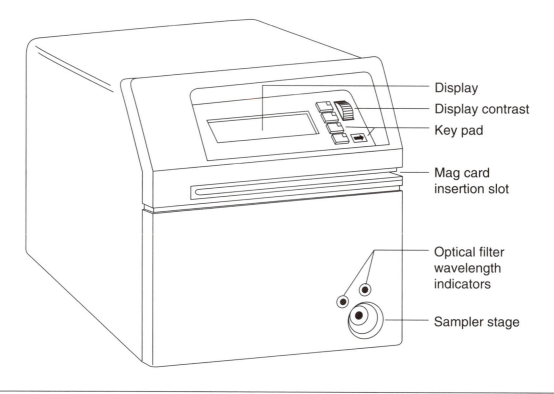

Display
Display contrast
Key pad
Mag card insertion slot
Optical filter wavelength indicators
Sampler stage

fig. 1.11. FIAX fluorometer

SUMMARY

Serology is the study of serum for antibody response to microorganisms, allergies, autoimmune diseases, and parasites.

The function of the immune system is to recognize foreign proteins and produce antibody against the protein for protection of the host.

There are two types of antigen response in a host. The first is cellular response, which is demonstrated by inflammation. The second is humoral response, which is the production of antibody.

Immunity can be passively or actively acquired. Immunity can also be acquired by artificial means.

Antigens are classified by their reactions either in vivo (in life) or in vitro (in a tube).

The five main classes of immunoglobulins are IgM, IgG, IgA, IgD, and IgE. The complement pathway is activated by IgM and IgG antibodies. The cells that influence the immune system are T and B lymphocytes.

Agglutination, precipitation, lysis, complement fixation, and inhibition are reactions seen most frequently in the serology laboratory.

Test procedures developed in the serology area use automated or semi-automated equipment. These procedures use fluorescence, ELISA, and flow cytometry.

REVIEW QUESTIONS

1. Define immunology.
2. Foreign proteins producing an immune response are
   a. lysozymes
   b. macrophages
   c. antigens
   d. antibodies
3. The main barrier to prevent invasion by foreign particles is
   a. lysozymes
   b. macrophages
   c. inflammation
   d. intact skin
4. Lysozymes are found in all of the following *except*
   a. tears
   b. stomach acid
   c. saliva
   d. mucosal membranes
5. Acute inflammation causes the formation of an/a
   a. exudate
   b. transudate

6. The fluid formed in inflammation contains
   a. fluid only
   b. cells only
   c. fluid and cells
   d. none of the above

7. The first cells to appear in an exudate are
   a. lymphocytes
   b. monocytes
   c. neutrophils
   d. eosinophils

8. The number of responses caused by penetration of a foreign agent into the body is
   a. five
   b. four
   c. three
   d. two

9. When a foreign agent penetrates the body, the response is
   a. humoral
   b. cellular

10. The production of antibody to an invading organism is
    a. humoral
    b. cellular

11. Antibody found in the serum of a neonate is
    a. passive acquired
    b. active acquired
    c. both a and b
    d. neither a nor b

12. Antibody formed after a disease process is
    a. passive acquired immunity
    b. active acquired immunity
    c. both a and b
    d. neither a nor b

13. The substance produced by the invasion of a foreign protein is
    a. antigen
    b. antibody
    c. complement

14. There are how many main classes of immunoglobulins?

15. Which portion of antibody is capable of binding antigen?
    a. Fab
    b. Fc
    c. hinge

16. Which portion of the antibody is responsible for antibody binding to monocytes?

17. Which portion of the antibody activates the complement pathway?
    a. Fab
    b. Fc
    c. hinge
18. The most abundant immunoglobulin found in serum is
    a. IgM
    b. IgG
    c. IgA
    d. IgE
19. The first immunoglobulin to appear after invasion of a foreign protein is
    a. IgD
    b. IgE
    c. IgM
    d. IgG
20. The second immunoglobulin to appear after invasion of a foreign protein is
    a. IgD
    b. IgE
    c. IgM
    d. IgG
21. The immunoglobulin that appears in great quantity to a second exposure to an antigen is
    a. IgD
    b. IgE
    c. IgM
    d. IgG
22. Which antibody is associated with allergic reactions?
    a. IgM
    b. IgG
    c. IgD
    d. IgE
23. Which immunoglobulin can be found on the surface of lymphocytes?
    a. IgM
    b. IgG
    c. IgD
    d. IgE
24. Which cells of the immune system are matured in the thymus?
25. Which cells of the immune system are formed in the bone marrow?
26. For the classical pathway of complement to be activated, which of the following must be present?
    a. calcium and magnesium
    b. calcium and potassium
    c. magnesium and chloride
    d. chloride and potassium

27. Which of the following antigens stimulates antibody formation and reacts in a visible manner?
    a. hapten(e)
    b. particulate
    c. soluble
    d. complete

28. Which antigen demonstrates complement fixation in an in vitro reaction?
    a. hapten(e)
    b. particulate
    c. soluble
    d. complete

29. Which antigen results in agglutination or lysis of test particles?
    a. hapten(e)
    b. particulate
    c. soluble
    d. complete

30. Which of the following is an incomplete antigen?
    a. hapten(e)
    b. particulate
    c. soluble
    d. all of the above

31. Agglutination reactions result in
    a. flocculation
    b. complement fixation
    c. lysis
    d. clumps

32. Precipitation reactions result in
    a. flocculation
    b. complement fixation
    c. lysis
    d. clumps

33. Lysis reactions result in
    a. flocculation
    b. cellular breakdown
    c. clumps
    d. complement fixation

34. What will an agar gel plate subjected to an electrical current form if an antigen-antibody reaction has taken place?

35. Immunoassay procedures use
    a. red blood cells
    b. complement
    c. enzymes
    d. all of the above

FURTHER ACTIVITIES

Have the students research literature on the preparation of vaccines and discuss the use of each vaccine researched.

Research and discuss electrophoretic patterns in disease processes.

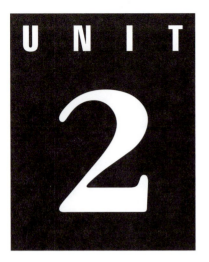

Safety Procedures and Quality Assurance

LEARNING OBJECTIVES

After studying this unit, the student should know the following objectives:

- Demonstrate proper hand washing.

- Demonstrate proper removal of soiled gloves.

- Identify pipettes used in serology.

- Demonstrate accurate pipetting.

- Prepare hypochlorite solution and discuss its use in the clinical laboratory.

- Discuss proper disposal of biohazardous material.

- Discuss proper use of the centrifuge and demonstrate proper methods of centrifugation.

- Discuss regulations dictating quality control procedures.

GLOSSARY

Acquired immune deficiency syndrome (AIDS): caused by the human immunodeficiency virus (HIV).

Autoclave: Equipment to sterilize by steam under pressure.

Biohazard: Name for any infectious material that presents a risk to health.

CAP: College of American Pathologists.

CDC: Centers for Disease Control and Prevention.

FDA: Federal Drug Administration.

Hepatitis: Inflammation of the liver.

JCAHO: Joint Commission on Accreditation of Hospitals and Organizations.

Microliter: One millionth of 1 L (µl).

Milliliter: One thousandth of 1 L (ml).

Nosocomial infection: Hospital-acquired infection.

OSHA: Occupational Safety and Health Administration.

Pipettes: Tubes used to transport and dispense small amounts of liquid.

Quality assurance: Program designed to evaluate and correct procedures in the laboratory.

Soluble: Capable of being dissolved.

Tuberculosis: Disease caused by mycobacteria.

Universal Precautions: Safety policies for handling biological specimens.

INTRODUCTION

People working in any area of health care must be safety conscious for their protection, as well as for the patients they are caring for. The laboratory worker must be very safety conscious due to the nature of the specimens that are processed in the laboratory every day.

Every laboratory has a set of instructions. These instructions may be titled standard operating procedures (SOPs) or operating instructions (OIs). Each laboratory will have its own particular title for this set of instructions.

SEROLOGY SAFETY PROCEDURES OVERVIEW

The Occupational Safety and Health Administration (**OSHA**) and the Centers for Disease Control and Prevention (**CDC**) write the safety and procedural guidelines for laboratory workers. These guidelines are called **universal precautions**. Common sense and adherence to the rules must be followed to prevent contamination to yourself, your fellow workers, and patients.

Because laboratory workers can carry microorganisms from person to person, patients in the hospital are often infected by hospital personnel not following universal precautions. The development of a disease process while in the hospital due to inadvertant infection with microorganisms is termed a **nosocomial infection**. The patient did not enter the hospital with the disease but has contracted the disease while in the hospital.

All infectious agents must be guarded against by laboratory workers. **Hepatitis, acquired immune deficiency syndrome (AIDS),** and **tuberculosis** are prevalent diseases and can be contracted by laboratory personnel. Laboratory personnel can contract any disease process they come in contact with at any time. All patient specimens must be handled as if they contain a communicable disease.

It is important to follow universal precautions and wear gloves at all times while handling patient specimens.

Every laboratory has printed guidelines for safety. It is important that you read and follow these instructions before you begin work in the area.

Quality assurance programs are necessary to evaluate the test procedures being performed and to correct any problems that may arise, either in the test or with the equipment being used.

Personal safety is very important. Laboratory coats and gloves must be worn when handling body fluids. Everyone should remember that it is possible for gloves to have minute holes, and these can let fluids reach the hands. Masks and goggles, or face shields, should be worn when appropriate.

The most important way to prevent cross contamination and the spread of disease is **hand washing.** It is very important to wash your hands after removal of gloves and before leaving the laboratory area. Laboratory coats should **never** be worn outside of the laboratory.

At no time should anyone eat, drink, smoke, or apply cosmetics in the work area of the laboratory. Hands should be washed before any of these activities.

It is recommended that all health care workers be immunized against hepatitis B virus.

EXERCISE 7 HAND WASHING

Have each student practice hand washing.

1. Stand in front of the sink. Do not lean on the sink with clothes. The front of the sink is considered contaminated.
2. Use a paper towel to cover the water controls and turn on the water. Adjust to warm temperature. Very hot water may irritate the skin and cause minute surface breaks.
3. Wet hands thoroughly. Hold hands lower than elbows so the water flows from arms to finger tips.
4. Apply soap to hands.
5. Wash the palm, back, and wrist of each hand using strong, frictional, circular movements. Avoid vigorous rubbing that could irritate the skin.
6. Interlace the fingers and thumbs. Move the hands back and forth for 15 seconds. This will remove organisms from the inside of the fingers.
7. Rinse the hands well. Allow water to flow from wrists to fingertips.
8. Dry hands thoroughly with a paper towel.
9. Use the paper towel to turn the water off. Do not soil hands by touching dirty water controls.
10. Put on gloves. There is no special technique for this procedure. Be careful not to tear gloves.

EXERCISE 8 SOILED GLOVE REMOVAL

Have each student practice removing his or her soiled gloves.

1. Grasp the glove to be removed on the palm side of your hand just below the cuff, being careful not to touch the bare skin on your wrist.
2. Pull the glove off by rolling it inside out. As you continue to hold the rolled-up glove with your fingers of the gloved hand, place the two fingers of your bare hand inside the cuff of the second glove.
3. Pull the second glove off by turning it inside out over the first glove.
4. Touching only the inside surface of the glove removed in step no. 3, dispose of the gloves in the appropriate container.
5. Wash your hands

ELECTRICAL SAFETY

Electrical shocks in the laboratory are a potential hazard. Electrical cords for equipment should never be exposed to any fluid. There should always be adequate electrical outlets for all equipment. Electric circuits must not be overloaded. Circuit overloads are potential fire hazards. *Do not use water on an electrical fire!*

FIRE SAFETY

All items for use in case of a fire are well marked. These items consist of fire blankets and fire extinguishers. Fire blankets are usually enclosed in a bright red metal container that is wall mounted. These blankets should be used if a person's clothing catches fire. Never attempt to extinguish a clothing fire with water. Always smother the flames with a blanket.

Several types of fire extinguishers are available. Some are used for paper fires, others for electrical fires or chemical fires. One class of extinguisher is used for all types of fire.

Every facility has an evacuation route to be used in case of fire or any emergency that would cause the evacuation of the laboratory. It is important to know that route. It could save your life.

EYE WASH STATION

Each laboratory is equipped with an eye wash station. It is important to know how to use the station in case of an accidental splash. Eye contamination happens in spite of universal precautions.

SAFETY SHOWERS

Safety showers are to be used in case of an accidental acid or biohazardous spill on clothing. It is important to know how to use the shower in case of an emergency.

CENTRIFUGES

Several types of centrifuges are used in the serology department. Angle head centrifuges are those that hold the tubes in a fixed position. Horizontal centrifuges

---

E X E R C I S E 9 SAFETY DISCUSSION AND DEMONSTRATION

Have the class
1. Discuss fire safety.
2. Research and discuss types of fire extinguishers.
3. Discuss evacuation routes and have students follow the route.
4. Demonstrate the use of a fire blanket.
5. Demonstrate the use of the eye wash system.
6. Demonstrate the use of the emergency shower.

swing the tubes to a horizontal position while spinning but return the tubes to a vertical position when they stop.

Centrifuge directions usually are given as revolutions per minute (rpm). Centrifuges generate a force when operating expressed as rcf (relative centrifugal force); rcf is sometimes referred to as G force.

Centrifuges come in two models. One model sets on the counter top, the other on the floor. They are referred to as tabletop and floor models. All centrifuges must have a cover on them to prevent aerosols from entering the environment.

General laboratory centrifuges attain speeds of 3,000 rpm for horizontal models and up to 7,000 rpm for angle head models.

Certain rules must be followed when one is working with centrifuges.

1. *Always follow the instructions for rpm and time of centrifugation.* Most tubes to be spun will have a speed and time given by the serology operating instructions (e.g., spin 10 minutes at 2,500 rpm).
2. Check the centrifuge cups to *be sure rubber cushions are in the cups.* Do not place tubes in cups if the rubber cushions are gone. If the cushions are missing, the tubes can break and the centrifuge will not be properly balanced.
3. *Be sure the tubes are balanced.* There should be the same amount in tubes placed across from each other in the centrifuge. To balance the centrifuge, you can use the same size tube filled with tap water.
4. *Do not remove caps from tubes before centrifuging.* Balance tubes should be capped also. If tubes are not capped, an aerosol can be created that increases the risk of infection to laboratory personnel.
5. *Keep the top of the centrifuge closed while in operation.* If a tube should break, the cover will prevent broken glass or the contents of the tube from flying out. The cover will also prevent aerosols from escaping into the air before the centrifuge rotor has stopped.
6. *Do not open the centrifuge until the rotor has come to a complete stop.* Do not lift the cover and attempt to stop the rotor with your fingers.
7. If a tube breaks in the centrifuge, *clean the centrifuge using universal precautions* before the centrifuge is used again.

BIOHAZARDOUS MATERIALS

Any material contaminated with body fluid is considered to be a **biohazard.** The contaminated materials must be placed in the proper containers for cleaning or disposal.

DISPOSAL METHODS

1. All nondisposable pipettes should be soaked in a 10% bleach solution (hypochlorite) between washings. All disposable pipettes should be disposed of in the proper containers with a biohazard symbol on the container.
2. Paper or gauze that is contaminated with body fluids should be placed in a container that is marked biohazard so it can be either incinerated or autoclaved. The containers for biohazardous waste are marked with a universal biohazard symbol (Figure 2.1). The bags will be either orange or red.

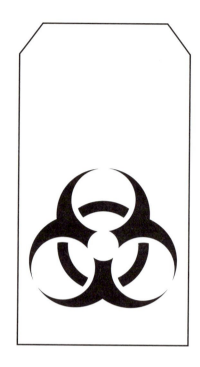

fig. 2.1. Biohazard symbol

3. When the contaminated bags are full, they must be placed in another bio-hazard bag. This is termed double bagging. The bags must be securely fastened at the top. If the material is to be picked up from the facility by licensed, contracted agencies for disposal, there must be a sticker attached to indicate the name and address of the facility generating the biohazardous waste.

4. There are special containers for broken glass and sharps. Sharps are defined as all material with sharp or jagged edges, such as needles, syringes, lancets, pipettes, broken glass, and slides. These containers are rigid and disposable and are marked with the biohazard symbol.

BASIC METHODS FOR WASTE DISPOSAL

1. Flushing down the drain. Anything flushed down the drain must be fol-lowed by large amounts of water and the drains periodically flushed with hypochlorite solution.
   The following items can be flushed down the drain:
   a. Blood from automated equipment
   b. Suctioned fluids
   c. Excretions (urine)
   d. Acids or bases after neutralization

2. Autoclaving. Some facilities use an **autoclave** for all materials generated by the laboratory.
   a. Microbiology specimens
   b. Pathology waste (from surgical specimens)
   c. Blood specimens or blood products

3. Incineration. Cotton balls or gauze contaminated with blood or body fluids may be incinerated.
4. Material that is not contaminated should be placed in regular waste receptacles for routine disposal. It is important to keep the contaminated material separated from the noncontaminated material. Most facilities hire companies to dispose of contaminated material for them. It is not cost effective for the facility to have the company dispose of noncontaminated material.

SPLASH SHIELDS

Splash shields are devices that set on the work counter (Figure 2.2). All tubes should be opened under one of these shields. When the cap is removed from a tube of body fluid, the cap should always be opened so that the bottom of the cap is away from the face. A shield will prevent body fluid from splashing on the face or in the eyes of the individual opening the tube.

Face shields, as well as splash shields, are also available in some facilities. This is a plastic shield that is held on the head by a band around the back of the head.

OTHER CONSIDERATIONS

Cuts or abrasions on the hands should be covered with a dressing before putting on gloves.

Work areas *must* be kept clean at all times. The area should be cleaned at the beginning and end of the work day. You cannot assume that the person you are replacing on a shift has cleaned the work area. All spills should be cleaned immediately.

The solution most commonly used to clean the work area is 10% hypochlorite solution (household bleach). Gloves should be worn when you are cleaning the work area.

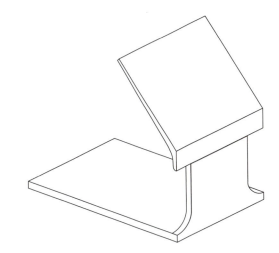

fig. 2.2. Splash shield

E X E R C I S E ▌10▐ SOLUTION PREPARATION

Have all students prepare 10% hypochlorite solution daily.

1. Measure 10 **ml** of bleach into a graduated cylinder (Figure 2.3).
2. Add 90 ml of water. Cover and mix well.

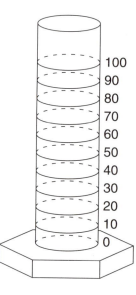

fig. 2.3. Graduated cylinder

PIPETTES

Many kinds of **pipettes** are used in the clinical laboratory (Figure 2.4), but our main focus is on the type of pipettes used in the serology section. *Never pipette by mouth!*

The most common type of pipette used in serology is called a serological pipette. It has a large tip opening and is designed to deliver fluids rapidly. The pipette is graduated to the end of the delivery tip and has an etched band on the top suction part. It is designed to be a "blow out" pipette. "Blow out" indicates that all liquid in the pipette must be expelled from the pipette. The unit of measurement used is the **milliliter** (ml).

Another type of pipette is a micropipette. This is a very precise pipette. It is a "to contain" pipette. "To contain" means it delivers the exact amount of fluid indicated by the size of the pipette. The unit of measurement used for micropipettes is the **microliter** (µl). The tips of the micropipette must be disposed of in a biohazard container after use.

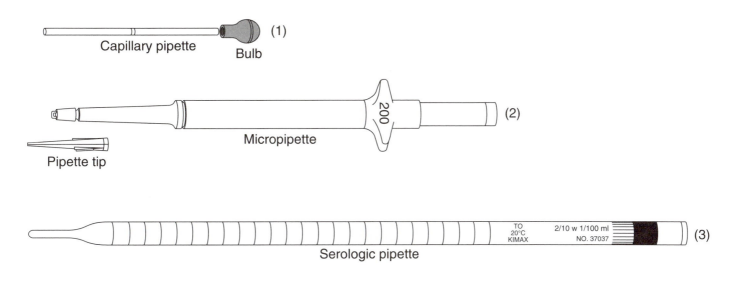

fig. 2.4. Pipettes

E X E R C I S E **11** **PIPETTE PRACTICE**

Have each student identify types of pipettes and practice pipetting with available pipetting devices.

1. Identify the pipettes used in serology.
2. Pipette 0.2 ml of water with a 0.2-ml pipette.
3. Pipette 0.2 ml of water and dispense 0.02, 0.04, and 0.08 ml.
4. Practice pipetting with 5- and 10-ml pipettes.

Capillary pipettes are the third type found in the serology laboratory. These pipettes are small glass tubes with a calibration line etched on the tube. These pipettes are marked for specified volumes. The pipette is filled by capillary action, and a small bulb is placed over one end to expel the fluid. This type of pipette is included in different serological test kits. This pipette must be disposed of in a biohazardous container for sharps.

More types of pipettes are used in other areas in the laboratory. The previously mentioned pipettes are the most common ones found in the serology department.

To use serological pipettes, one must use a device to aspirate the fluid being measured (Figure 2.5). Many types of aspirators are used in the laboratory. Some are large bulbs; others are cylinders with a thumb ratchet. These devices must be used with serological pipettes to fill the pipette with fluid. When one is pipetting, the meniscus of the fluid should be on the top mark of the pipette (Figure 2.6).

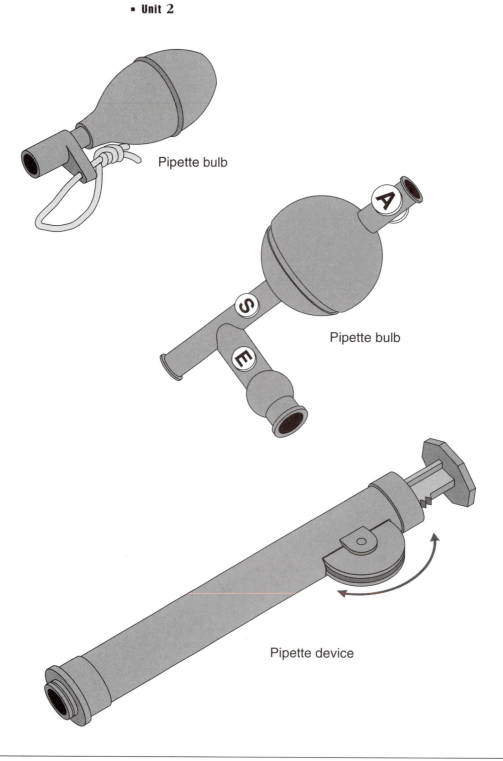

Pipette bulb

Pipette bulb

Pipette device

fig. 2.5. Aspirating devices

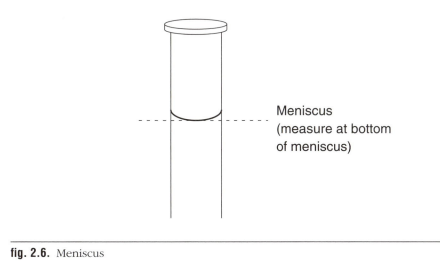

Meniscus
(measure at bottom
of meniscus)

fig. 2.6. Meniscus

DAILY QUALITY ASSURANCE

HEAT BLOCKS AND WATER BATHS

All heat blocks and water baths must contain a thermometer that has been calibrated against a National Biological Standards (NBS) thermometer. The thermometer's calibration must be performed before use and periodically thereafter.

The temperature of the heat block well must be read and recorded each working shift. To read the temperature of the heat block, place a tube containing fluid, either water or saline solution, in the well. The thermometer is placed in the tube. The readings of the well are taken during each shift for 24 hours.

The tube with the thermometer is then moved to the next well and the procedure repeated until each well has been checked for temperature. The thermometer should read ±0.5°C for the set temperature of the heat block. One set of heat blocks should be set for 37°C and one set for 56°C.

Water bath temperatures are also read and recorded each working shift. The temperature of the water baths are usually set at 37°C and 56°C. Water baths usually have a holder for the thermometer. The water should be moving when the temperature is read.

REFRIGERATION TEMPERATURES

Many laboratory refrigerators are equipped with internal and external temperature reading devices and recorders. The refrigeration temperature range is 4°C to 6°C. Readings must be taken from the external chart and compared with the reading from the internal device. Most refrigerators with internal monitoring devices have a probe that must be kept in a solution of glycerine water to simulate the temperature at which liquids must be maintained. A thermometer is kept in the liquid and must be read and recorded each working shift. The inside thermometer must equal or nearly equal, within a fraction of a degree, to the outside recording device.

The temperatures of both monitoring systems must be read and recorded each shift.

Note: If the refrigerator has a "power out" monitoring alarm, the alarm must be checked weekly by allowing the temperature of the refrigerator to warm above the highest temperature setting.

A notation must be made in the record for the temperature at which the alarm rang. The temperature is then cooled below the lowest setting, and again a notation must be made when the alarm rings.

All temperature readings when the alarm rings must be written in the quality assurance log with the date and initials of the person performing the test.

REAGENT TEST KITS

All test kits contain positive and negative controls. These controls must be performed with each battery of tests in compliance with the manufacturer's instructions.

The test kits also contain lot numbers and expiration dates. These data must also be included in the daily quality assurance log for the test kits.

When new test kits are opened, the new reagents should be tested against both the controls in the kit being opened and against the controls of the kit that no longer contains reagent. This is a check on the reactivity of both controls. Some lot number kits have weaker reacting controls than others. The strength of the control aids the technician or technologist evaluating the test results. This double check of controls must be placed in the quality assurance log with the lot numbers being tested, the date of the test, and the initials of the person performing the test.

Never mix reagents from different kits. Use only the reagents in the test kit that is opened.

The date on which test kits are opened should be annotated on the kit with the initials of the person opening the kit. This information is part of the quality assurance log.

Kits used for testing with automated and semiautomated equipment will have a set of standardized controls with assayed amounts of antigen or antibody, depending on the test procedure. These controls must be performed with the battery of tests on the day performed. A record of the control readings must be maintained in the quality assurance log for each test, the lot number of the kit, the date of test, and the initials of the person performing the testing.

Rotators for RPR (rapid plasma reagin) or VDRL (Venereal Disease Research Laboratory) testing must be tested on the day of use (see Unit 3, p. 55). The number of rotations per minute must be made and recorded, also the date of the test and the initials of the person performing the test.

MONTHLY QUALITY ASSURANCE

CENTRIFUGES

Centrifuges must be calibrated monthly. The revolutions per minute must be checked with a tachometer, and the timer must be checked with a stopwatch. If the number of revolutions per minute or the timer do not meet manufacturer specifications, the equipment must be repaired before continuing use.

Centrifuges have brushes in the centrifuge mechanism. These brushes wear out over time and must be replaced by the maintenance department.

A quality assurance log must be maintained for the number of revolutions per minute, timer check, and any maintenance performed on the equipment. Dates and initials of the person performing the check must be on the log.

Stopwatches used for the timer check must also be calibrated. One way to perform this check is to dial a toll-free telephone number in Denver and calibrate by the atomic clock.

Even though it seems repetitive to perform the quality assurance checks and balances, it is necessary to do so. Accreditation of each area of the laboratory is necessary to continue the operation of the departments.

In hospitals, inspections to accredit the laboratory are conducted by the College of American Pathologists **(CAP),** the Joint Commission of Hospital Accreditation and Organizations **(JCAHO),** and the Federal Drug Administration **(FDA).** Accurate records are a necessity to pass the inspections, maintain accreditation, and continue to be able to function.

Each quarter (every three months), laboratories receive from the CAP specimens for testing in each section of the laboratory. The test results must be accurate to maintain accreditation. This is an external quality assurance evaluation.

Each laboratory sets up internal quality assurance checks and balances to assure that reagents and equipment are within set parameters. It is also a check on the performance of personnel.

SUMMARY

Following the guidelines of **OSHA** and the **CDC** and practicing universal precautions are instrumental in preventing contamination of yourself and your co-workers.

These precautions will aid in preventing nosocomial infections during patient care.

The use of the proper cleaning solutions and care in disposal of contaminated material is necessary to prevent the spread of communicable diseases through the laboratory.

Using the proper pipettes and properly disposing of the pipettes will aid in protection for you and your co-workers. The proper use of pipetting devices and accuracy in pipetting are also important. Practice is the key to accuracy.

Proper disposal of all biohazardous material is of primary importance and must comply with state and national regulations.

The most important way to prevent bacterial or viral contamination to yourself or to those around you is *hand washing.*

In all areas of the laboratory there must be a system in operation to assure that reagents give the desired results and have not lost reactivity. This system is known as quality control or quality assurance.

Equipment must be maintained by both the laboratory and the maintenance department to assure it is operating to manufacturer specifications.

Records must be kept on all reagents and equipment. The records must contain the date of testing, test results, and the name of the individual or individuals who have performed the testing.

Quality assurance programs are necessary to maintain accreditation of the facility. It also assures that the personnel will be able to continue to work.

The bottom line when one is using equipment, reagents, and kits is to read the manufacturer's instructions and follow the instructions completely.

REVIEW QUESTIONS

1. The guidelines for laboratory safety are written by
   a. NCCLS and OSHA
   b. NCCLS and CDC
   c. CDC and OSHA
   d. all of the above

2. Laboratory guidelines should be read
   a. before working in the laboratory department
   b. when you have time
   c. because the supervisor requires reading
   d. to keep your job

3. Handling body fluids requires the technician to wear
   a. gloves
   b. lab coat
   c. gloves or lab coat
   d. gloves and lab coat

4. The most *important* way to prevent spreading disease is to
   a. wear gloves
   b. wear a lab coat
   c. wash hands frequently
   d. use a splash shield

5. Water temperature for washing hands should be
   a. warm
   b. cold
   c. hot
   d. any of the above

6. To remove organisms from between the fingers the hands should be washed
   a. 5 seconds
   b. 15 seconds
   c. 30 seconds
   d. 45 seconds

7. The solution most commonly used to clean the work area in the laboratory is
   a. 10% phenol
   b. 10% bleach
   c. 5% Lysol
   d. 5% formalin

8. The pipettes used in the serology laboratory are
   1. serological
   2. micropipettes
   3. capillary
   4. volumetric

      a. 1 and 2

      b. 2 and 4

      c. 1, 2 and 3

      d. 4 only

9. A centrifuge may be opened
   a. after the rotor comes to a complete stop
   b. when the rotor slows down
   c. anytime during centrifugation
   d. all of the above

10. Paper towels used to dry hands should be placed in a biohazard container.
    a. true
    b. false

11. Sharps are defined to include
    a. broken glass
    b. lancets
    c. needles
    d. all of the above

12. Which of the following *should not* be flushed down the drain?
    a. blood
    b. microbiology specimens
    c. suctioned fluids
    d. neutralized acids

13. A splash shield will protect the technician's
    a. hands
    b. eyes
    c. hands and eyes
    d. eyes and face

14. Cuts or abrasions on the hands do not need to be covered if gloves are worn.
    a. true
    b. false

15. Caps should always be removed from tubes before centrifugation.
    a. true
    b. false

16. Quality assurance records must contain all of the following *except*
    a. date
    b. time
    c. results
    d. technician/technologist's initials

17. Controls on test kits must be performed
    a. weekly
    b. monthly
    c. daily
    d. yearly

18. Maintenance records on equipment do not have to be kept in a quality assurance log.
    a. true
    b. false

19. Internal and external quality assurance surveys are necessary to maintain accreditation.
    a. true
    b. false

20. Inspection agencies include all of the following *except*
    a. JCAHO
    b. CAP
    c. FDA
    d. ASCLS

FURTHER ACTIVITIES

Obtain a copy of *Universal Precautions,* published by the CDC in Atlanta.

Obtain a copy of the rules of your state on biohazardous waste disposal.

Write a quality assurance program for a serology department.

Write a safety manual for a serology department.

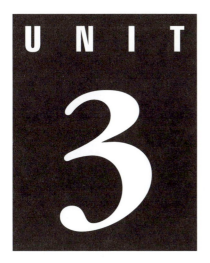

UNIT 3

Syphilis Serology

LEARNING OBJECTIVES

After studying this unit, the student should be able to:

◼ Discuss the physical manifestations of syphilis.

◼ Discuss other disease processes that produce a positive test result for syphilis.

◼ Differentiate the four stages of syphilis and discuss the clinical symptoms for each.

◼ Discuss the different nontreponemal and treponemal serological tests used in the diagnosis of syphilis.

◼ Explain the causes for false-positive and false-negative results in the RPR test.

◼ Discuss the quality control needed in the RPR test.

◼ Discuss the reagents in the RPR antigen and the action of each.

GLOSSARY

Cation: Ion with a positive electrical charge.

Chancre: A hard syphilitic primary ulcer.

Chelate: Use of a compound to bind to chemical ring structure.

Dark-field: Black background in microscopic field.

ELISA: Enzyme-linked immunosorbent assay.

FTA-ABS: Fluorescent treponemal antibody-absorption test for syphilis.

Genus: Taxonomic division between species and family.

Hemagglutination: Clumping of red blood cells.

Nonreactive: Negative reaction.

Nontreponemal antigen test: Serological test for antibody to syphilis without the treponemal antigen.

Pinta: Infectious skin disease caused by *Treponema carateum*.

Prozone reaction: An excess of antigen in a diluted serum that does not react in low dilutions but reacts in higher dilutions.

Qualitative: Presence of product (antibody) in serum.

Quantitative: Amount of product (antibody) in serum.

Reactive: Positive reaction.

Reagin: Antibody-like substance produced in response to the spirochete *Treponema pallidum*.

Rapid plasma reagin (RPR): Serological test for detection of reagin (antibody-like substance) produced in response to *Treponema pallidum*.

Spirochete: Slender, spiral, motile microorganism; any member of the order Spirochaetales.

TPHA: *Treponema pallidum* hemagglutination test.

TPI: *Treponema pallidum* immobilization test.

Treponemal antigen test: Procedure using treponemes in the test.

Treponema pallidum: Spirochete that is the causative agent of syphilis.

Treponemes: Organisms of the genus *Treponema*; another name for spirochetes.

VDRL: Venereal Disease Research Laboratory.

Yaws: Disease caused by *Treponema pertenue*.

INTRODUCTION

Syphilis, a contagious sexually transmitted disease, has been known for centuries. It is suspected that members of the royal families, as well as the commoners, in Europe had syphilis. Syphilis became a pandemic (worldwide) disease as explorers went from country to country.

Syphilis is spread mainly by sexual contact. The disease process is easier to detect in men than in women. Men will develop a penile lesion; in women the lesion will often be found only in the vagina. The lesion is not easily detected because of vaginal secretions normally present in the female. The female **chancre** can be anywhere in the genital area. The lesion can also be on the clitoris or the labia.

The early treatment for syphilis was administration of arsenical compounds. That treatment was often worse than the disease. Today penicillin is used to treat syphilis; however, some forms of the disease are penicillin resistant.

Syphilis is caused by the **spirochete *Treponema pallidum.*** This spirochete causes an immune response in the body. The antibody-like substance produced in plasma or serum is **reagin.** Reagin is the substance detected in a **nontreponemal antigen test.**

If syphilis is not treated, it progresses through four stages.

STAGES OF SYPHILIS

PRIMARY STAGE

Chancres or skin lesions appear at the site of the *T. pallidum* infection after an incubation period of approximately three weeks. The incubation period can be one week to three months before the chancre appears.

During the course of this stage, the infected person will develop enlarged lymph nodes and a chancre. If the fluid produced by the chancre is spread on a glass slide and examined with a **dark-field** microscope (a microscope with a condensor that darkens the background and causes the organism to appear white), the spirochete can be seen. The serological test result for syphilis will usually be **nonreactive** (negative) at this time.

Some of the organisms will remain at the infection site; others will be carried by the bloodstream to every organ in the body, causing systemic infection. The chancre will heal with or without treatment.

SECONDARY STAGE

The secondary stage of syphilis occurs from six to eight weeks after the appearance of the chancre. In this stage of the disease, the patient has fever, malaise, mucous patches in the mouth, and a generalized rash. Lesions may develop in the joints, eyes, or central nervous system. The rash will usually disappear within two to six weeks.

Dark-field examination of the fluid in the rash will still show the presence of *T. pallidum*. Serological test results at this stage become **reactive** (positive).

LATENT STAGE

After the second year of the infection, syphilis enters into the latent stage and is usually not contagious. In this stage there are no clinical symptoms, but serological test results are reactive. However, if spinal fluid is tested at this stage, the test result for syphilis will be nonreactive. This stage may last for several years or for the life of the person. If the infection has persisted for four years or more, it is rarely communicable. However, at this time, the disease can be transmitted from mother to fetus.

TERTIARY STAGE

The tertiary stage is referred to as late syphilis. Lesions can appear three to ten years after the primary stage. The lesions are located on the skin and mucous membranes. Lesions can also form in bones, joints, and muscles. The lesions are not infectious. If the lesions are present in the nervous system, the results of the lesions may cause blindness, paralysis, and other neurological problems.

Serological test results for syphilis may be reactive or nonreactive at this stage. If the nervous system is involved, the spinal fluid will usually give a reactive result.

If a pregnant woman is infected with syphilis, the organism is capable of crossing the placental barrier and infecting the fetus with syphilis. When the child is born, the test result for syphilis will be reactive. Some of these children will have a low titer of reagin for the rest of their lives. This type of syphilis is termed congenital syphilis.

Some individuals, after being treated for syphilis, will always have a low-titer reactive test result for syphilis. The term for this condition is seroconversion and indicates an antibody response to an antigen. These individuals are termed as being serofast.

NONVENEREAL SYPHILIS

Due to worldwide travel, it is important to learn about other types of treponemal disease that will cause a serological reactive test result for syphilis.

Treponema carateum is a common cause of the disease **pinta.** This disorder is found in Mexico, Venezuela, Columbia, India, and the Philippines. *Treponema carateum* will usually cause a false-positive test result for syphilis in the second stage of the disease process.

E X E R C I S E **12** **TREPONEMAL DISCUSSION**

Have the students discuss pinta and yaws.

1. Discuss clinical symptoms in pinta and yaws.
2. Discuss differences in clinical symptoms among pinta, yaws, and syphilis.

Treponema pertenue is the causative agent of **yaws.** This nonvenereal disease can be either acute or chronic and resembles syphilis. It does not involve the genital area. Yaws is typically a disease of childhood and is found in the Philippines, the Caribbean Islands, South America, and Africa.

NONTREPONEMAL ANTIGEN TESTS

VDRL SLIDE TEST

The VDRL (Venereal Disease Research Laboratory) test is a rapid slide microflocculation, nontreponemal serological test used as a screening test for syphilis. This test is read microscopically. It can be used for determining both the presence of reagin (qualitative) and the amount (quantitative) of reagin present in serum. It can be used as a follow-up after treatment for syphilis. If the therapy is effective, the antibody titer will decrease or become nonreactive.

The stock antigen for the VDRL test contains a colorless alcoholic solution of cardiolipin, lecithin, and cholesterol. To prepared working antigen, an aliquot of antigen is mixed with a buffered saline solution, pH 6.0, provided with the antigen by the manufacturer.

Plasma cannot be used for this test procedure.

VDRL QUALITATIVE AND QUANTITATIVE PROCEDURES

Both the quantitative and qualitative tests are performed the same. The only difference is that the serum in the quantitative test must be serially diluted. The dilutions are 1:1, 1:2, 1:4, and 1:8. The titer will be reported in dils (dilutions). For the quantitative VDRL, serial dilutions of the inactivated serum used for the qualitative test are used.

When titering any serum for antigen-antibody reactions (Figure 3.1), you must be aware of a **prozone reaction** (Figure 3.2). A prozone reaction is one in which there is an excess of antibody in the serum for the amount of antigen used. If a prozone reaction takes place, there will be no reaction in the tubes until the antibody in the serum has been diluted enough to be in equilibrium with the antigen. If the first well is negative when reading a titer, continue to read the rest of the wells to be certain a prozone reaction is not present.

INTERPRETATION OF RESULTS

A reactive result indicates the presence of reagin, which may not be produced by **treponemes** responsible for syphilis. This type of reaction is termed a biological false positive and may be caused by pregnancy, lupus, and other diseases or by technical error (Table 3.1).

SPINAL FLUID VDRL TEST

VDRL tests are performed on spinal fluid to detect the tertiary stage of syphilis. Spinal fluid must *not* be heated before testing. The antigen for the test procedure

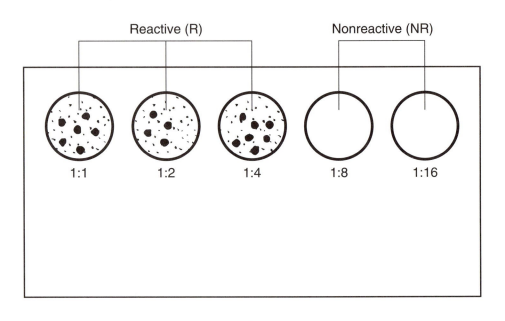

fig. 3.1. VDRL reactions

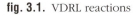

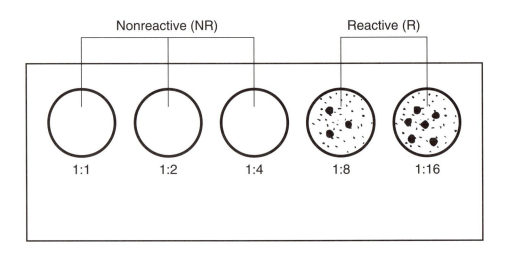

fig. 3.2. Prozone reaction

Table 3.1. Sources of Error in the Quantitative VDRL

1. Reagents not at room temperature. If they are too cold, there is a decrease in sensitivity; if they are too warm, there is an increase in sensitivity.
2. Cloudy serum containing particles.
3. Prozone reaction.
4. Antigen emulsion not well mixed.
5. pH changes in the buffer.
6. Stale antigen. Antigen must be used the day it is prepared.
7. Room temperature too hot or cold.

E X E R C I S E **13** **QUALITATIVE VDRL PROCEDURE**

Following the manufacturer's directions, assemble the materials needed to perform a qualitative VDRL:

VDRL stock antigen
Buffered saline solution (comes with the stock antigen)
Slide with 14-mm rings
Pipettes: 1 and 5 ml
18-gauge needle and a syringe
Mechanical rotator

A. Place the patient's serum into a 56°C heat block for 30 minutes.
B. Prepare the VDRL antigen as follows:
  1. Pipette 0.4 ml of buffered saline solution into a bottle with a flat bottom.
  2. Add 0.5 ml of VDRL antigen drop by drop while rotating the vial in a circular motion. Blow the last drop from the pipette.
  3. Add 4.1 ml of the buffered saline solution to the vial.
  4. Place the top on the bottle and shake back and forth approximately 30 times in 10 seconds. The antigen is now ready for use.
  5. Calibrate an 18-gauge needle attached to a syringe. The needle must deliver 60 drops/ml of antigen.
C. Procedure:
  1. Allow inactivated serum to cool to room temperature.
  2. Place 0.5 ml of inactivated serum into one of the 14-mm circles on the slide.
  3. Place 0.5 ml of positive control into one of the 14-mm circles on the slide.
  4. Place 0.5 ml of the weakly positive control into one of the 14-mm circles on the slide.
  5. Place 0.5 ml of the negative control into one of the 14-mm circles on the slide.
  6. Hold the syringe in a vertical position. Add one drop of the antigen suspension from the 18-gauge needle and syringe.
  7. Place the slide on the mechanical rotator. Rotate for eight minutes at 180 rpm.
  8. Examine each well microscopically with the low-power (10 X) objective.

Results:

Nonreactive—no clumping or slight roughness
Weakly reactive—small clumps
Reactive—medium to large clumps

Note: If the test is weakly reactive or reactive, a quantitative VDRL test must be performed.

EXERCISE 14 QUANTITATIVE VDRL PROCEDURE

Using a slide with 14-mm rings, prepare the serial dilutions as follows:

1. Pipette 0.05 ml of 0.90% saline solution into rings 2, 3, and 4 on the slide.
2. Pipette 0.05 ml of inactivated serum into rings 1 and 2.
3. Mix the saline-serum mixture in ring 2 and transfer 0.05 ml of the mixture from ring 2 to ring 3.
4. Mix the saline-serum mixture in ring 3 and transfer 0.05 ml of the mixture from ring 3 to ring 4 on the slide.
5. Aspirate 0.05 ml of the mixture from ring 4 and discard.
6. Add one drop of antigen to each well (1–4) from the calibrated 18-gauge needle and syringe. Hold the syringe in a vertical position.
7. Place the slide on the mechanical rotator and rotate the slide for eight minutes at 180 rpm.
8. Examine each well microscopically with the low-power (10 ×) objective.

must be diluted before use with 10% saline solution. The test is performed the same as the serum test.

RPR TESTING*

The most frequently performed nontreponemal test for syphilis is the **rapid plasma reagin (RPR)** test. It is less time consuming than the VDRL test and easier to perform.

The Macro-Vue RPR Card Tests are macroscopic, nontreponemal testing procedures for the serological detection of syphilis, which use unheated serum or plasma obtained from venous blood or blood collected by a finger puncture. The testing procedure is described in the *Manual of Tests for Syphilis*, published by the Centers for Disease Control, Atlanta.

The test techniques described are widely used in the United States and have been thoroughly evaluated and standardized. All materials employed in the RPR Card Tests are economical, disposable, and contained in compact kits occupying a minimum amount of space when stored or in use.

Each lot of RPR Card antigen is tested for conformance to Centers for Disease Control and Prevention (CDC) product specifications.

The 18-mm Circle RPR Card Test is the recommended test when venous blood collection is employed. To perform this test, one needs 0.05 ml of serum or plasma.

*The following information on the RPR card tests is reproduced with permission from BBL Microbiology Systems, a division of Becton Dickinson and Company, Cockeysville, Md.

Procedure. The RPR Card antigen suspension is a carbon-containing, cardiolipin antigen that detects reagin, which, as mentioned earlier, is an antibody-like substance present in the blood of syphilitic persons and occasionally found in the blood of individuals with other acute or chronic conditions. The RPR Card antigen suspension is prepared from stock VDRL antigen. When the VDRL antigen is added to buffered saline solution, lipid particles consisting of cholesterol coated with cardiolipin and lecithin are formed. The suspension of lipid particles is centrifuged to produce a sediment that is resuspended in a special fluid containing the disodium salt of ethylenediamine tetraacetic acid (EDTA), phosphates, thimerosal, choline chloride, and charcoal.

The EDTA enhances the stability of the suspension by inhibiting the oxidation or peroxidation of lipids, usually catalyzed by **cations.** One must complex or **chelate** the cations, if present, with EDTA. Charcoal acts as the visualizing agent. The phosphates buffer the suspension. Thimerosal acts as a preservative. Choline chloride serves as a chemical "inactivator" of inhibitors present in fresh serum or plasma, which prevent the agglutination of the lipid particles by reagin. These inhibitors are conventionally inactivated by heating. The presence of choline chloride eliminates the need for heat inactivation and makes possible the testing of unheated serum or plasma. However, heat inactivated serum samples can also be tested.

When the test is performed, the RPR Card antigen suspension (containing the lipid particles and finely divided charcoal particles) is mixed with the serum or plasma. If reagin is present, it will combine with the lipid particles, causing them to agglutinate. When this occurs, the finely divided charcoal particles are coagglutinated, resulting in black clumps of varying intensity, which are clearly visible against the white background of the plastic-coated cards. The specimen showing this result is reported as reactive. If reagin is absent, the lipid particles are not agglutinated, and the charcoal particles are not coagglutinated, resulting in an even gray color in the test mixture. The specimen showing this result is reported as nonreactive.

Antigen Precautions. The temperature of the testing area must be 23°C to 29°C, and all materials (including antigen) must be warmed to this temperature before testing. Immediate use of a refrigerated reagent will result in decreased sensitivity of the test.

The antigen suspension must not be used beyond the expiration date.

The RPR Card antigen should be tested on a daily basis with controls of predetermined reactivity before it is used to test clinical specimens.

Antigen Delivery. Gently resuspend the RPR card antigen by inverting the dispensing bottle several times before use. Holding the bottle in a vertical position, dispense approximately five drops into the dispensing bottle cap to make sure that the needle passage is clear. Then place one free-falling drop onto each test area. *Do not mix; the mixing of antigen suspension and specimen is accomplished during rotation.* Do not predrop on the card because this may be a source of contamination of the antigen in the recovery step.

Brewer Diagnostic Cards. The diagnostic test cards are specially prepared, plastic-coated cards that have been designed for use with the RPR Card Test procedures. In handling, care should be taken not to finger-mark the test areas on the card, because this may result in an oily deposit that will prevent proper spreading of the serum. *Do not use a soiled or bent card.* Each test area should be used only once. The card should be discarded after use (Figure 3.3).

Dispensing needles contained in the RPR Card Test kits are square cut and siliconized. The 20-gauge, yellow hub needle used with the 18-mm Circle RPR Card Tests dispenses $\frac{1}{60}$ ml of antigen per drop.

To maintain clear passage of the needle for accurate drop delivery, on completion of the daily tests, remove the needle from the dispensing bottle and rinse it with distilled or deionized water, shake it to remove excess moisture, and replace it in its protective shield. Do not wipe the needle, because this will remove the silicone coating and may affect the accuracy of the drop of antigen being dispensed.

When each new kit is opened, the accuracy of the needle contained therein should be checked. Check delivery of the needle by placing the needle firmly on a l-ml pipette; fill the pipette with antigen suspension, and, holding the pipette in a vertical position, count the number of drops delivered in 0.5 ml. The correct number of drops should be 30 ± 1 drop.

Rotator. The Macro-Vue Card Test Rotator is specifically designed for use with the RPR Card Tests. It circumscribes a circle 2 cm in diameter in a horizontal plane. The 127 × 177.8 mm rotator top conveniently accommodates two qualitative cards or one large quantitative card. The neoprene covering guards against card slippage and can be easily cleaned. Placement of the timer dial is such that the eight-minute setting required for RPR Card testing is clearly visible.

The recommended speed of rotation is 100 rpm, but rotation between 95 and 110 rpm does not significantly affect the results obtained. At less than 95 rpm and more than 110 rpm, the clumping of antigen tends to be less intense in tests with undiluted serum, so that some minimal reactions may be missed. In quantitation, rotation greater than 110 rpm tends to produce an approximately one-dilution decrease in titer.

To check the rotator speed, hold a pen next to the rotating platform and count the number of taps per minute.

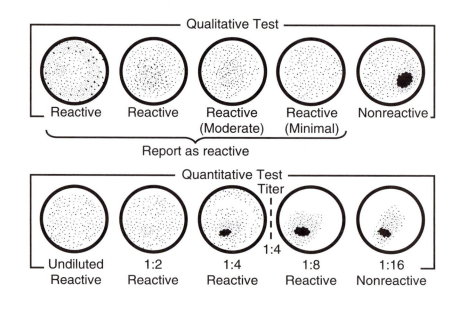

fig. 3.3. RPR 18-mm reactions

Humidifying Cover. A humidifying cover is provided with each Macro-Vue Card Test Rotator (Figure 3.4). It is used to minimize evaporation and ensure that all tests are conducted under the same level of humidity to achieve uniform results.

For use, saturate the absorbent material in the handle with approximately 10 ml of water. Add water from time to time to maintain the humidifying effect.

Periodically remove the absorbent material, clean thoroughly, and rinse with a disinfectant solution to prevent microbial growth.

Testing Area. The temperature of the testing area must be 23°C to 29°C, and all materials must be warmed to this temperature (room temperature) before testing. If the area is too warm, the incidence of false-positive reactions will increase. If the area is too cold, the sensitivity of the test will decrease, and false-negative test results and less intense reactions will be produced. The testing area, if possible, should be well lighted, clean, and free from drafts.

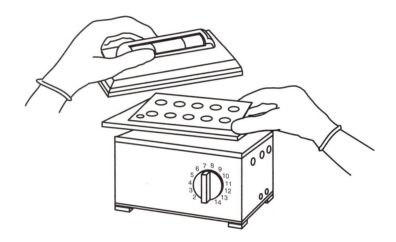

fig. 3.4. Rotator with humidifying cover

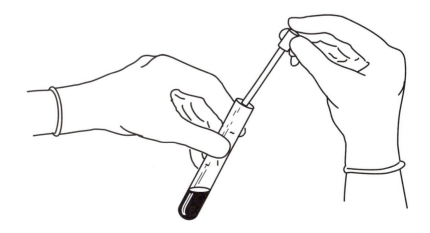

fig. 3.5. Holding Dispenstirs device

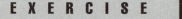

E X E R C I S E   **15**   **18-MM CIRCLE, QUALITATIVE RPR CARD TEST USING DISPENSTIRS**

Following the manufacturer's instructions

1. Calibrate the 20-gauge needle.
2. Prepare the control cards for testing.
3. Hold the Dispenstirs device between the thumb and forefinger near the stirring or sealed end (Figure 3.5). Squeeze and do not release pressure until the open end is below the surface of the specimen, holding the specimen tube vertically to minimize stirring up cellular elements when using the original blood collection tube. Release finger pressure to draw up the sample.
4. Holding the Dispenstirs device in a vertical position directly over the card test area to which the specimen is to be delivered, squeeze the Dispenstirs device, allowing one drop to fall on the card (approximately 0.05 ml).
5. Invert the Dispenstir device and spread the specimen to fill the entire circle. Discard the Dispenstir device. Repeat the procedure for each specimen to be tested.
6. Gently resuspend the RPR card antigen several times. Place one drop of antigen on each of the test areas. *Do not mix.*
7. Rotate the card for eight minutes under a humidifying cover on a mechanical rotator at 100 rpm.
8. After rotation, tilt the card by hand three or four times. Then immediately read macroscopically under a high-intensity lamp or in strong daylight.
9. Report as reactive, showing characteristic clumping ranging from slight but definite to marked and intense; or nonreactive, showing slight roughness or no clumping.

Note: There are only two possible reports with the RPR Card Test: *reactive* (regardless of the degree of clumping) or *nonreactive.*

Reactive minimal to moderate (showing slight, but definite clumping) is always reported as reactive.

All reactive results should be confirmed by retesting the specimen using the quantitative procedure. Some common causes of incorrect results and their solutions can be found in Table 3.2.

The RPR Card Test qualitative method can be performed using capillary pipettes designed to deliver 0.05.

Record results as nonreactive or reactive.

A quantitative RPR test procedure can be performed to determine the titer of reagin in the serum or plasma.

EXERCISE 16 **QUANTITATIVE RPR TESTING**

Following the manufacturer's directions, assemble all materials needed to perform the 18-mm Circle, Quantitative RPR card test (machine rotation).

Use 0.05-ml capillary pipettes or a 50-lambda pipetting device for quantitation.

1. For each specimen to be tested, place 0.05 ml of 0.9% saline solution onto the circles numbered 2 to 5. A marked capillary pipette, a serological pipette, 1 ml or less, or pipetting device may be used. *Do not spread saline solution!*

2. Using a capillary pipette with a rubber bulb attached or a pipetting device, place 0.05 ml of specimen into circle 1.

3. Refill the capillary pipette to the red line or pipette tip with the test specimen. Holding it in a vertical position, place the specimen onto circle 2 and prepare serial twofold dilutions by drawing the mixture up and down five or six times. Avoid the formation of bubbles. Transfer 0.05 ml from circle 2 to 3, 3 to 4, 4 to 5, etc. Discard 0.05 ml after mixing the contents on circle 5.

4. Using a clean stirrer (broad end) for each specimen, start at the highest dilution of serum (circle 5) and spread the serum to fill the entire circle to, but not beyond, its periphery. Proceed to circles 4, 3, 2, and 1 and accomplish similar spreading.

5. Gently resuspend the RPR Card antigen by inverting the dispensing bottle several times before use. Holding the bottle in a vertical position, dispense approximately five drops into the dispensing bottle cap to make sure that the needle passage is clear. Then place one free-falling drop (20-gauge, yellow hub needle) of antigen ($\frac{1}{60}$ ml) onto each test area. Do not mix; mixing of antigen suspension and specimen is accomplished during rotation. Pick up the predropped antigen from the bottle cap.

6. Rotate for eight minutes under a humidifying cover on a mechanical rotator at 100 rpm. After mechanical rotation, to help differentiate nonreactive from reactive results, briefly rotate and tilt the card by hand. Then immediately read *macroscopically* in the "wet" state under a high-intensity lamp or in strong daylight.

Report in terms of the highest dilution giving a minimal-to-moderate reaction.

Table 3.2. Troubleshooting the RPR Test

FALSE NEGATIVE	FALSE POSITIVE	QUANTITATION TOO LOW	QUANTITATION TOO HIGH
1. Rotator malfunction	1. Serum allowed to dry before antigen is added.	1. Improper dilution	1. Insufficient amount of saline solution
2. Excess serum	2. Rotated too long	2. Air bubbles	2. Starting the mixing process at highest reagin content and progressing to the lowest reagin content.
3. Insufficient or excess amount of antigen	3. Rotated under no cover or a dry cover	3. Excess saline solution	
4. Cold reagents	4. Excessive high temperature of reagents	4. Insufficient amount of serum	
5. Cold room temperature	5. Excessively high room temperature	5. Improper amount of antigen	
6. Outdated antigen	6. Reading error	6. Reading error	
7. Excess agitation of antigen	7. Rough antigen	7. Excess serum	
8. Insensitive antigen		8. Excess antigen	
9. Reading error			

TREPONEMAL ANTIGEN TESTING

Treponemal antigen testing uses either live or dead *T. pallidum* to determine the presence of antibodies to the *T. pallidum* spirochete.

One of the first tests used for the detection of syphilis was the Wasserman test. This is a complement fixation test, which is seldom, if ever, used today. It was a lengthy, tedious test. Other complement fixations tests are Reiter's Protein Complement Fixation and Treponemal Pallidum Cryolysis Reaction. Because of the complexity of these tests, they are no longer used in the serology laboratory.

TREPONEMAL PALLIDUM IMMOBILIZATION TESTS

In *T. pallidum* immobilization **(TPI)** tests, the patient's serum is placed on a slide or in a tube with live spirochetes from infected rabbit tissue and complement. The test is incubated in an anaerobic atmosphere, and a portion of this serum-spirochete mixture is placed on a slide and examined using dark-field microscopy. If the serum is from a person with syphilis the spirochetes will be immobilized. If the serum does not contain antibodies from a syphilitic patient, the *T. pallidum* spirochetes will be motile.

This test procedure will rule out biological false-positive reactions caused by other microorganisms.

FLUORESCENT TREPONEMAL ANTIBODY–ABSORPTION TEST

In the fluorescent treponemal antibody–absorption **(FTA-ABS)** test the patient's serum is reacted with dead *T. pallidum* on a slide or in a test tube. The material is then incubated with anti–human globulin, which has been mixed with a dye (fluorescein). If the antibodies to *T. pallidum* are present in the serum, the *T. pallidum* spirochete will fluoresce. If there is no fluorescence, the test result is negative. A special type of microscope must be used for this test.

TREPONEMA PALLIDUM HEMAGGLUTINATION TEST

The *T. pallidum* **hemagglutination (TPHA)** test is a recent addition for syphilis testing. It has replaced the FTA-ABS procedure in many laboratories. In the TPHA procedure, tanned sheep cells are coated with antigen from Nichol's strain of *T. pallidum*. The serum is absorbed with a sorbent. The red blood cells will agglutinate if antibodies for syphilis are present in the serum.

ENZYME-LINKED IMMUNOSORBENT ASSAY

In the enzyme-linked immunosorbent assay **(ELISA)**, the inside of tubes are coated with *T. pallidum* antigen. Patient serum is added to the tubes, which are then incubated. The tubes are washed after the incubation period, and an enzyme-labeled anti–human globulin is added. Substrates are added to the tube. The amount of enzyme activity is measured by a colorometric method.

SUMMARY

Syphilis is a disease spread mainly by sexual contact, although it can be transmitted from mother to fetus in utero.

Syphilis, if untreated, progresses through four stages: primary, secondary, latent, and tertiary.

Other diseases, such as pinta and yaws, can result in a biological false positive for syphilis. These disease processes are called nonvenereal syphilis.

The test procedures to detect the antibody-like substance (reagin) in the serum of patients with syphilis are nontreponemal antigen tests. The VDRL test is performed mainly on cerebral spinal fluid to detect the tertiary stage of syphilis.

The test procedure routinely used for serological testing is the RPR. It is an easy test to perform, and either plasma or serum can be used for testing purposes.

Other test procedures for the detection of syphilis are treponemal antigen tests, such as TPI tests, the FTA-ABS test, the TPHA test, and ELISA.

REVIEW QUESTIONS

1. Syphilis is caused by
   a. *Treponema pertenue*
   b. *Treponema carateum*
   c. *Treponema pallidum*
   d. Herpes simplex
2. A treponeme is a
   a. spirochete
   b. cocci
   c. bacillus
   d. virus

3. The third stage of syphilis is
    a. secondary
    b. latent
    c. tertiary
    d. primary

4. The syphilitic rash appears in the what stage of syphilis?
    a. primary
    b. secondary
    c. latent
    d. tertiary

5. The material from a syphilitic chancre is examined by
    a. phase microscopy
    b. bright field
    c. polarized light
    d. dark field

6. In which untreated stage of syphilis is the RPR test result reactive?
    a. primary
    b. secondary
    c. latent
    d. tertiary

7. Central nervous system involvement appears in which stage of untreated syphilis?
    a. primary
    b. secondary
    c. tertiary
    d. latent

8. In the VDRL test for syphilis the term reactive indicates a
    a. positive test reaction
    b. negative test reaction

9. A prozone reaction is a(an)
    a. antigen excess
    b. antibody excess
    c. nonreactive test result
    d. minimal reactive test result

10. The VDRL and RPR are
    a. treponemal tests
    b. nontreponemal tests

11. The RPR test is performed on
    a. plasma
    b. serum
    c. whole blood
    d. both a and b

12. Choline chloride in the RPR antigen acts as a
    a   chemical inactivator
    b. visualizing agent
    c. preservative
    d. stabilizer

13. Charcoal in the RPR antigen acts as a
    a. chemical inactivator
    b. visualizing agent
    c. preservative
    d. stabilizer
14. The RPR test is rotated at how many rpms?
    a. 200
    b. 180
    c. 100
    d. 80
15. The RPR test is rotated for how many minutes?
    a. 4
    b. 6
    c. 8
    d. 10
16. All of the following will cause a false-negative RPR result *except*
    a. excess serum
    b. cold reagents
    c. outdated antigen
    d. room temperature too warm
17. All of the following will cause a false-positive RPR test result *except*
    a. rough antigen
    b. rotated too long
    c. rotated without a cover
    d. cold reagents
18. Treponemal antigen tests use
    a. live *T. pallidum*
    b. dead *T. pallidum*
    c. both a and b
    d. neither a nor b
19. Live spirochetes are used in which of the following tests?
    a. ELISA
    b. TPI
    c. FTA-ABS
    d. TPHA
20. Tanned sheep cells are used in which of the following tests?
    a. ELISA
    b. TPI
    c. FTA-ABS
    d. TPHA

FURTHER ACTIVITIES

Write to the CDC and order the *Manual of Tests for Syphilis,* 1969, PHS Publication No. 411.

Visit a public health laboratory and observe testing for syphilis by TPHA, FTA-ABS, ELISA, or available procedures.

Divide the students into groups and have them discuss the following:

1. TPI tests
2. TPHA tests
3. FTA-ABS
4. ELISA methods

UNIT 4

Viral Diseases

After studying the unit, the student should be able to do the following:

- Discuss the viral types of hepatitis.

- Discuss the types of test procedures that differentiate the types of hepatitis.

- Explain why pregnant women should not be immunized.

- Name the three types of heterophil antibodies.

- List the types of test procedures used to identify infectious mononucleosis.

- Discuss the stages of acquired immunodeficiency syndrome (AIDS).

- List the types of test procedures used to diagnose AIDS.

- List the types of test procedures to detect cytomegaloviruses.

GLOSSARY

Acute: Having rapid onset.

AIDS: Acquired immunodeficiency syndrome.

Chronic: Of long duration.

CMV: Cytomegalovirus.

Counterelectrophoresis: Process in which antigens and antibodies are placed in separate wells and an electric current is passed through the diffusion medium.

HAV: Hepatitis A virus.

HBsAg: Hepatitis B surface antigen.

Hepatitis: Inflammation of the liver.

Heterophil(e): An antibody reacting to other than a specific antigen.

NANB hepatitis: Non-A, non-B form of hepatitis.

Opportunistic infections: Infections resulting from a defective immune system.

Rubella: Acute infectious disease, commonly called German measles.

Surrogate tests: One test replacing another.

INTRODUCTION

Viruses are the smallest protein agents that produce disease. Viruses are also called virions. This term is used to indicate the complete viral particle.

Viruses have only DNA or RNA, not both, as do other microorganisms. Viruses must infect living tissue to be able to reproduce; they are considered to be parasites.

Viruses are usually classified by the diseases they produce, such as **hepatitis** (inflammation of the liver).

The viruses that will be discussed in this unit are hepadnavirus (hepatitis), togavirus **(rubella),** herpesviruses (infectious mononucleosis [IM] and cytomegalovirus [CMV]) and retrovirus (acquired immunodeficiency syndrome [AIDS]).

As just mentioned, hepatitis is a term used to indicate an inflammation of the liver. The liver can become inflamed by many processes (virus, bacteria, parasites, drugs, or alcohol). In serology laboratories great emphasis is placed on hepatitis to determine if the condition is the result of viral contact.

Viral hepatitis is a communicable disease that is found worldwide. Hepatitis is more commonly found in areas with poor water quality and poor sanitation.

The first identification of the hepatitis virus was found in the serum of a group of people living in Australia. The virus was named "Australia antigen." This virus was later classified as hepatitis B.

The viruses associated with hepatitis are viral hepatitis A **(HAV),** viral hepatitis B (HBV), Non-A, Non-B hepatitis **(NANB hepatitis),** and viral hepatitis D (HDV). Other viruses associated with hepatitis are Epstein-Barr virus (EBV), rubella, and cytomegalovirus (CMV), among others. Several of these viruses will be discussed in this unit.

A patient with viral hepatitis will have a variety of clinical symptoms, including low-grade fever, fatigue, malaise, anorexia, nausea, and vomiting. The skin will become yellow, or jaundiced, as will the eyeballs. The patient's urine will become dark yellow, and the feces will become clay colored.

Due to the number of symptoms that are similar to other diseases, it is hard for the physician to diagnose without ordering specific test procedures. One of the orders will be for a hepatitis battery of tests, along with, possibly, a test for IM.

The role of the laboratory is to supply the physician with laboratory results to aid in the diagnosis of the patient's disease.

HEPATITIS A VIRUS

The hepatitus A virus (HAV) incubates approximately 14 to 42 days. In the infectious stage the virus is highly contagious. It is spread by the fecal-oral route. It is transmitted by contaminated food and water. The virus is excreted in the feces during the infectious stage.

There is evidence of an increased incidence of HAV in child care centers and orphanages. In adults HAV is usually associated with contaminated food. Raw oysters are a contaminant for humans due to the contaminated water from which the shellfish are taken.

The symptoms are mild in HAV, with recovery in 7 to 21 days. However, there are cases that last for one year or more.

There are enzyme immunoassay (EIA) tests for HAV to detect both the antigen and the antibody.

HEPATITIS B VIRUS

The hepatitus B virus (HBV) is known as "serum hepatitis," or hepatitis B surface antigen **(HBsAg).** This virus is transmitted via blood transfusions, sharing dirty needles among drug users, and via sexual intercourse.

The incubation time for the virus is 30 to 180 days. The virus is found in blood and body secretions. The virus is carried via infected blood, saliva, and semen. It can enter the body through small breaks in the skin or can be transmitted during sexual intercourse if there is a break in the mucous membrane.

Individuals who are immunosuppressed are at risk of contracting HBV (e.g., multiple-unit transfused patients, hemophiliacs on cryoprecipitate therapy, dialysis patients, renal transplant patients, intravenous drug users, and individuals with leukemia). All health care personnel are at risk if they handle needles or body fluids of patients with hepatitis.

Mothers who are HBV carriers can transmit the virus to their infants during the birth process.

Mandatory screening of all donor blood for hepatitis has made the blood supply safer.

The HBV infection can become **chronic.** The individual can become a carrier or develop chronic hepatitis. The carrier state is defined as HBsAg in the blood for six months with normal liver function test results. Individuals with chronic hepatitis are divided into two categories.

The first category is called chronic persistent hepatitis. The patient in this category will have abnormal liver function test results with a normal liver biopsy specimen.

The second category is called chronic active hepatitis. These patients have abnormal liver function test results and abnormal liver biopsy specimens.

Clinical laboratory tests ordered in suspected cases of hepatitis are performed on serum and are called liver function tests. These tests are performed in the chemistry department. The tests are bilirubin, alanine aminotransferase (ALT), and aspartate transaminase (AST). The ALT and AST are liver enzyme tests.

In **acute** hepatitis the transaminase levels rise markedly. The transaminase level rises sharply in HAV infections and slowly in HBV and in non-A, non-B (NANB) hepatitis infections. Bilirubin levels rise in viral hepatitis infections. Other chemical tests ordered on serum are albumin and globulin. In hepatitis the serum albumin level is decreased and the serum globulin level is elevated.

The HBV appears in three forms: (1) spherical particle; (2) filamentous form; and (3) Dane particle, which is least commonly found in the patient's blood.

Hepatitis B markers are: (1) HBsAg, outer lipoprotein coat; (2) HBcAg, core antigen of HBV; and (3) HBeAg (Figure 4.1).

The HBeAg is found during the acute phase. If it persists past the acute phase, it is an indication of chronic hepatitis.

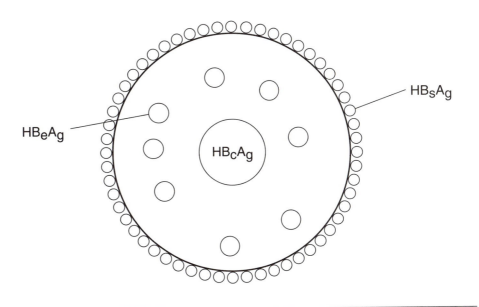

fig. 4.1. Dane particle

HEPATITIS D VIRUS

The hepatitus D virus (HDV) is also called "delta hepatitis." The patient must have HBV present to acquire HDV. The HDV needs the outer envelope of the HBV to reproduce and produce a clinical disease.

NON-A, NON-B HEPATITIS

This type of hepatitis is just what the name indicates. It is neither HAV nor HBV. There is little knowledge as to the exact cause of non-A, non-B (NANB) hepatitis. It is the most common type of hepatitis caused by transfusions. Blood banks are required to perform chemical tests called **surrogate tests.** These surrogate tests are markers for HBsAg. The ALT (a liver enzyme test) and anti-HBc (antibody to the core antigen of HBV test) do not identify the same markers, so both must be performed. The NANB hepatitis contains hepatitis C, which can become a chronic condition.

Hepatitis E virus has been found, but at this time a test has not been developed to screen for the virus.

The test procedures devised for testing of hepatitis were given names as the procedures became more sophisticated.

GENERATION TESTS

The first-generation tests were performed on Ouchterlony agar gel plates (Figure 4.2). The test itself took a very short time to set up, but the results took 24 hours. The antibody for the HBsAg was put in the plate in one well. Patient's serum was

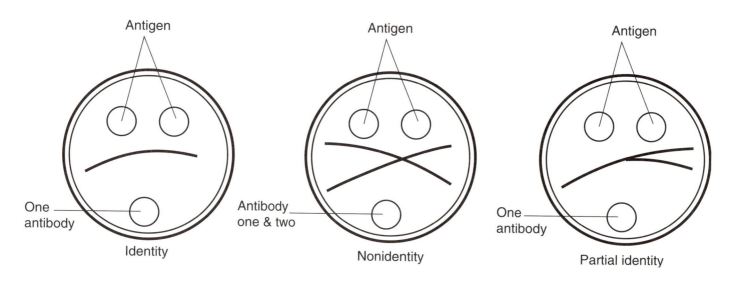

fig. 4.2. Ouchterlony agar plate

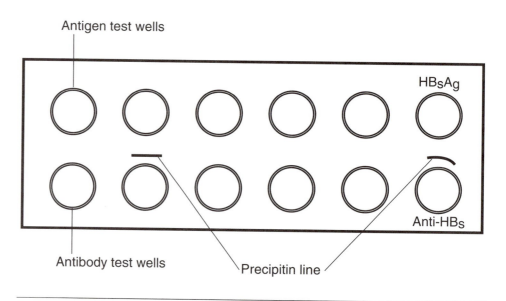

fig. 4.3. Counterelectrophoresis

placed in the wells surrounding the antibody. If the test result was positive, there was a fine white precipitin line formed between the antigen and antibody. The test was not very sensitive.

A second-generation test commonly used for HBsAg was **counterelectrophoresis** (Figure 4.3). The antibody was placed in wells of an agar plate across from wells containing patient serum. The plates were subjected to an electric current. If the antigen was in the serum, a fine precipitin line would form.

Third-generation test procedures consist of radioimmunoassay (RIA) and enzyme-linked immunoassay (ELISA, one of the common EIA tests). Other test procedures in the third generation were reverse passive hemagglutination and reverse passive latex agglutination tests.

E X E R C I S E   **17**   HEPATITIS MARKERS

Have the students prepare a chart for the serological markers for

1. The acute stages of hepatitis.
2. The chronic stages of hepatitis.

The ELISA is replacing the other third-generation tests. The ELISA procedures can be automated and used for batch testing. This assay also eliminates the problem of radioactive material disposal, which is a problem with RIA.

RUBELLA

Rubella at one time was a common disease. With the advent of rubella vaccines, mass immunizations of children, and the routine vaccination of infants, there has been a decrease of cases in the Western world.

Rubella is also called German measles. Rubella begins as an upper respiratory tract infection with enlarged lymph nodes and a skin rash.

The rash will appear approximately 14 days after exposure to the rubella virus. Antibodies to rubella will appear at this time. The antibody test result for rubella will become positive after the first week. The titer of antibody will rise for two weeks and then begin to decline. The titer will be positive for years, or there will be a low titer that will last a lifetime.

The IgM and IgG antibody elevations in rubella parallel each other, which does not happen in other viral diseases. In other disease processes, IgM antibody is produced and then IgG antibody is produced.

The rubella virus in pregnant women can cross the placenta and affect the fetus. If this occurs, the infant may be born severely affected with congenital heart defects, deafness, or brain damage.

A test for rubella is one of the tests performed in the prenatal patient test battery.

A pregnant woman exposed to rubella should have her immune status tested if this has not been done previously. If she has a significant titer of antibodies within 10 days after exposure, she usually is immune. A second blood specimen should be drawn two to four weeks after exposure to determine if there is a rise in titer. If an IgM antibody titer is performed approximately three weeks after exposure and the titer is elevated, it is an indication of a recent infection.

A fetus exposed to the rubella virus in utero can produce both IgM and IgG antibodies. The fetus can also have maternal IgG antibody to rubella.

The maternal IgG antibody will disappear from the newborn within six to eight months. If the antibody remains in the serum longer, it is an indication of fetal infection.

TESTS FOR RUBELLA ANTIBODY

Hemagglutination tests (Figure 4.4), latex agglutination, and ELISA are test procedures used to determine the presence of the rubella antibody. As with other procedures, ELISA is becoming the test of choice.

Individuals who have been exposed to rubella must have two blood specimens drawn. The specimens are usually obtained two weeks apart. There should be a fourfold rise in titer from the first to second specimen if the patient has IgM antibodies. The two sera are tested together. When two sera from the same individual are to be tested with the same procedure, the specimens are referred to as paired specimens. After the first specimen is tested, it is frozen and retested when the second specimen is drawn.

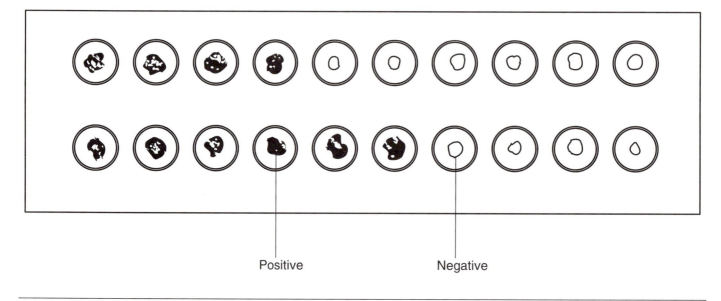

Positive   Negative

fig. 4.4. Passive hemagglutination

CASE STUDY

Have the class discuss the following:

On a prenatal visit, a woman who is two months pregnant tells her physician that one of her children has rubella. Her other children are not immunized. The pregnant woman did not have a titer for rubella on her first prenatal visit.

Should the doctor be concerned that the other children and the pregnant women are at risk of contracting rubella? Should the children be immunized? Should the pregnant woman be immunized at this time?

INTERPRETATION

The presence of antibody in a patient's serum is an indication that the patient has been infected with the rubella virus or the patient has had a rubella immunization.

The children who were not immunized have been exposed to the rubella virus. Immunization at this time may or may not prevent the onset of rubella in the children. There is always a chance that a pregnant woman can contract rubella from a child or anyone else who has recently had a rubella immunization. The virus is shed in saliva and feces. Rubella immunizations are usually not given to pregnant women due to the makeup of the vaccines that are administered.

INFECTIOUS MONONUCLEOSIS

Infectious mononucleosis (IM) is caused by Epstein-Barr virus (EBV). The EBV is a human herpesvirus. The immunoglobulin associated with the disease is IgM. The antibody is one of the heterophile antibodies (Table 4.1). It is an acute disease of the reticuloendothelial system. This disease is prevalent in the teen years to the middle to late twenties and is commonly called the "kissing disease." Another name for the disease is "glandular fever." It is thought that the disease is transmitted from person to person by saliva. The virus actually infects the B lymphocytes. The name mononucleosis has no connection with the monocyte in the white blood cell series. "Mono" in this case means "one" and "nucleosis" refers to the cell nucleus. Lymphocytes have one nucleus.

The clinical findings are similar to other types of diseases previously discussed. The patient complains of fatigue, low-grade fever, swollen glands, and a sore throat. On examination the doctor finds splenomegaly (enlarged spleen) and hepatomegaly (enlarged liver). Some patients have a jaundiced or yellow color to the skin.

Laboratory findings show atypical or reactive lymphocytes and elevated liver function enzyme test results.

SEROLOGICAL TESTS

The IM **heterophil(e)** antibodies are the IgM type. They appear the first week of the illness and peak about the third to fourth week. The antibody level will begin to decline after the fourth week and become undetectable thereafter.

Several types of test procedures are available for the detection of IM antibodies in serum. One of the first procedures was the Paul-Bunnell test.

The Paul-Bunnell test required that a serial dilution of heat-inactivated serum be prepared. Heat-inactivated serum has been heated at 56°C for 30 minutes. A

Table 4.1. Types of Heterophil(e) Antibodies

1. Forssman—antibodies produced as a result of incidental contact with antigens unrelated to the individual species. Almost everyone has heterophile antibodies to the Forssman antigen in a low titer in the serum.
2. Serum sickness—antibody produced to injection of vaccines that were prepared from horse serum. This type of antibody is rarely seen because of the modern preparations of vaccines.
3. IM—antibody produced in response to EBV.

2% saline suspension of sheep cells was added to the tubes. The tubes set at room temperature for 2 hours and then were examined for agglutination. Heterophile antibodies of the IM variety would agglutinate sheep cells. Because a titer of 1:28 is normal, a titer of 1:56 or more was diagnostic of IM infection. This test is termed a presumptive test because it was found that other heterophile antibodies would also agglutinate sheep cells.

The next test developed was the Davidsohn Differential Test. This test used guinea pig kidney and beef erythrocytes. Guinea pig kidney is a good source of Forssman antigen and will combine with Forssman antibodies. The IM heterophile antibody is not absorbed by guinea pig kidney. The IM antibody is absorbed by beef erythrocytes, but the Forssman antibody is not absorbed.

Laboratories now use other types of testing, usually termed "spot" tests (Figure 4.5). These tests use the same principles as the Paul-Bunnell and Davidsohn tests but are performed on a slide. A titration is not usually performed if the spot test results are positive. However, the test kits usually will have a procedure for titration if the procedure is requested by the physician.

The spot tests use horse erythrocytes in place of sheep cells as the antigen. Guinea pig kidney antigen is used in these procedures as in the Davidsohn differential. In these test procedures, an aliquot of serum is mixed with beef erythrocyte antigen on one side of a slide and guinea pig kidney on the other side of the slide. Horse erythrocytes are added to each side of the slide and mixed. If the serum-cell mixture with guinea pig kidney antigen agglutinates, the serum is positive for IM antibodies. If no agglutination occurs, the test result is negative for IM antibodies. Positive and negative controls are included in the test kit and must be performed with the tests each time the tests are performed.

One of the newer tests on the market uses EIA membrane technology for the determination of IM antibody in serum or plasma.

Other tests on the market place all reactants on cards provided in the kit. The patient's serum is added to the spot on the card, mixed, and observed for agglutination.

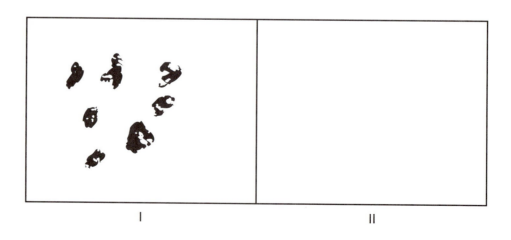

I   II

fig. 4.5. Spot test

EXERCISE **18** SPOT TEST FOR INFECTIOUS MONONUCLEOSIS

Following the manufacturer's instructions, perform a test for IM.

1. Place the slide that comes with the kit on a flat surface under a light source.
2. Invert the cells contained in the kit several times. Using a microcapillary pipette provided in the kit, place one drop of the cells to one corner of both squares on the slide.
3. Place one drop of thoroughly mixed reagent I to the center of square I.
4. Place one drop of thoroughly mixed reagent II to the center of square II.
5. Add one drop of the serum being tested into the drops of reagent in squares I and II.
6. Mix the reagent and serum in each square thoroughly (8–10 times). Do not blend in the cells at this time.
7. Stir the reagent-serum mixture into the cells and spread over the entire surface of each square on the slide.
8. *Do not move the slide*.
9. Observe for agglutination for no longer than one minute after mixing.

Interpretation

If the agglutination is stronger in square I, the test result is *positive*. If the agglutination is stronger in square II, the test result is *negative*. If there is no agglutination in either square I or II, the test result is *negative*. If there is equal agglutination on both sides, the test result is *negative*.

ACQUIRED IMMUNODEFICIENCY SYNDROME

Acquired Immunodeficiency Syndrome (AIDS) is one of the most destructive human diseases to appear since the great plagues in the Middle Ages.

In the United States, the disease was first discovered in homosexual men; therefore, it was thought of as a disease affecting only homosexuals. It later was found in heterosexual men and women. Persons with hemophilia developed the disease due to their requirements for factor VIII (coagulation factor) to stop bleeding episodes. Factor VIII is found normally in human plasma. The disease was transmitted to hemophiliacs via infusion of cryoprecipitate, which is rich in factor VIII.

This disease is transmitted by sexual contact, transfusion of blood and blood products, and miscellaneous infection through the use of dirty needles and syringes by drug users. Health care providers are at risk due to needle sticks and accidental splash of body fluids. *Remember that gloves are not impervious to needle punctures*. The virus can be transmitted if there is a break in the skin or mucous membrane and an accidental splash of blood or other body secretions gets into the open area. The virus has been found in semen, vaginal secretions, saliva, tears, breast milk, amniotic fluid, urine, and cerebrospinal fluid.

Many infants are infected with the AIDS virus at birth from an AIDS-positive mother.

The causative agent of AIDS is the human T-cell-trophic retrovirus type III. This virus is also called the human immunodeficiency virus (HIV) and lymphadenopathy-associated virus (LAV).

In the early stages of HIV infection, which may last for months, the patient may be asymptomatic or demonstrate a mild flu-like syndrome, with fever and a skin rash. There may or may not be a swelling in the lymph nodes. At this time the antibody to HIV will appear. Some patients may be symptom free for years, but in other patients the disease progresses rapidly, and the patient has a very short life span.

As the immune system is weakened by the AIDS virus, the patient will have other opportunistic diseases, such as hepatitis, cytomegalovirus (CMV), *Pneumocystis carinii* pneumonia, tuberculosis, and Kaposi's sarcoma.

The virus attaches to cells in the body that have a protein receptor site called CD4. The viral RNA invades the cell's cytoplasm, where the virus replicates itself (Figure 4.6). When the cell divides, the virus is transferred with the new cell.

The cells affected by HIV are T lymphocytes. In healthy persons T cells (helper cells) outnumber suppressor cells in a 2 to 1 ratio. People with AIDS have the reverse. Suppressor cells outnumber T cells, leaving the person with a weakened or an ineffective immune system. When the immune system is weakened or becomes ineffective, the virus and other **opportunistic infections** are able to affect the patient.

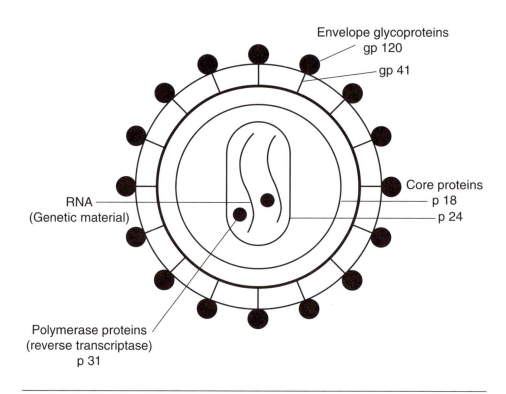

fig. 4.6. AIDS virus

Many test procedures can detect the AIDS antibody. One of the test procedures used is the EIA test. This test is performed using microwells or beads coated with antigenic preparations of inactivated and lysed whole virus. The patient's serum is incubated with the bead and will react with the immunosorbent if antibody is present. The bead is then washed, and an enzyme-conjugated second antibody specific for human immunoglobulin is added and allowed to react with bound antibody. The bead is washed, and a substrate is added. The color change is measured spectrophotometrically. This color change is compared with a standard of known concentration and is directly proportional to the amount of HIV-1 antibody present in the patient's serum. If this test result is positive, it is followed by another test to confirm the presence of the HIV antibody. The second test is a Western Blot test.

The Western Blot test is performed by separating the HIV proteins by molecular weight into discrete bands. This is done by electrophoresis onto polyacrylamide gels. The proteins are then moved onto nitrocellular sheets and cut into strips. The strips are incubated overnight with the patient's serum. The strips are then washed and incubated with antihuman immunoglobulin that has been conjugated with enzymes or biotin. After the substrate has been added, color will develop to show discrete bands when antigen-antibody reactions have occurred.

Test results are considered positive when the gp41 band appears alone or when an envelope antibody (gp41, gp120, or gp160) is in combination with another HIV band (p15, p18, p24, gp41, p51, p55, p66, gp120, or gp160). The test result is considered negative if there is no appearance of bands.

Other methods have been devised for HIV testing, such as immunofluorescence assay, immunohistochemical staining, ELISA, RIA, and polymerase chain reaction (PCR).

Test results can be negative for the antibody due to a certain time period called a "window" phase when neither the antigen nor the antibody to the AIDS virus can be detected in serum.

All units of blood drawn in the United States are tested for HIV. If test results for a unit are positive, it is destroyed.

CYTOMEGALOVIRUS

Cytomegaloviruses (CMVs) are herpesviruses that cause human disease. The virus may be transmitted from person to person by close contact with viral material. The incubation period ranges from 28 to 56 days in children and adults. The disease mimics infectious mononucleosis (IM). The disease process is called cytomegalic inclusion disease.

The virus can cause lifelong infections. The virus can be shed from the pharynx and in the urine. The virus is species specific. Animal CMVs exist but will not infect humans. Conversely, human CMVs will not infect animals.

The CMV usually does not cause severe disease process in the immunocompetent host. However, the immunosupressed host is at great risk for CMV. The persons at greatest risk are those receiving organ transplants, AIDS patients, and patients who are on chemotherapy for malignancies. The most common complication in these patients is pneumonia.

If CMV is present in a pregnant woman, she can transmit the disease to the fetus. Many of the babies born with CMV will have developmental defects and mental retardation. The virus can be acquired by the infant from the birth canal by exposure to the virus in the mother's genital tract during delivery. The virus can also be acquired from breast milk.

Antibodies to CMV occur frequently in human serum. The antibodies are of the IgM, IgG, and IgA classes.

Antibodies in the serum may be detected by immunofluorescence tests, RIA, or complement fixation.

SUMMARY

Viruses are the smallest protein agents that produce diseases in humans. They are parasitic and must have living tissue in which to reproduce. The viruses most commonly tested for in the serology laboratory are Epstein-Barr (EBV) (IM antibody), hepatitis, rubella, cytomegalovirus (CMV), and acquired immunodeficiency syndrom (AIDS).

There are several types of hepatitis: HBsAg, called serum hepatitis due to the route of infection; hepatitis A virus (HAV), transmitted by the fecal-oral route; and non-A non-B hepatitis (NANB), of which little is known as to the exact cause of this type of hepatitis.

Rubella is a virus responsible for measles. Children in day-care centers are often infected with this virus if they have not been protected against the disease. Pregnant women who have not had measles or the vaccine are at risk of infecting the fetus if they are exposed to rubella or have an active infection. The infant can be born with hearing difficulties, and mental retardation, and in some cases the infant will be stillborn.

Infectious mononucleosis (IM) is a disease of the young, often called the kissing disease. The causative agent of IM is EBV. The virus affects the B lymphocytes.

AIDS is one of the most destructive human diseases. It is found in all classes of people, including homosexuals, heterosexuals, the young, the old, men, and women. The disease process destroys the immune system and leads to opportunistic infections and, ultimately, death.

CMV is a herpesvirus that may cause human disease. In the immunocompetent system the virus usually remains quiescent, but it will manifest itself in the immunosupressed as CMV. This virus is capable of crossing the placental barrier and infecting the unborn fetus. The infant can be born with developmental defects and mental retardation.

REVIEW QUESTIONS

1. Hepatitis is an inflammation of the
   a. heart
   b. lungs
   c. stomach
   d. liver

2. Another name for serum hepatitis is
   a. hepatitis B surface antigen
   b. hepatitis A
   c. Non-A, Non-B
   d. hepatitis D

3. The route of transmission for hepatitis A is by
   a. blood
   b. contaminated food
   c. contaminated water
   d. b and c

4. HBV carriers can transmit the virus to their infant during the birth process.
   a. true
   b. false

5. All of the following are liver function tests *except*
   a. ALT
   b. AST
   c. glucose
   d. bilirubin

6. Which of the following is an indication of chronic hepatitis?
   a. HBeAg
   b. HBsAg
   c. HAV
   d. both a and c

7. Rubella commonly affects which age group?
   a. infants
   b. pre teens
   c. middle aged adults
   d. geriatric adults

8. Another name for rubella is
   a. German measles
   b. three-day measles
   c. rubeola
   d. a and c

9. Rubella virus can cross the placental barrier and affect the fetus.
   a. true
   b. false

10. The fetus exposed in utero can produce
    a. IgA
    b. IgM
    c. IgG
    d. both b and c

11. The causative agent of IM is
    a. rubella
    b. rubeola
    c. EBV
    d. CMV

12. In the spot test for IM, the cells used in the procedure are
    a. guinea pig
    b. horse
    c. sheep
    d. goat
13. What lymphocyte is decreased in the immunosuppressed patient?
14. The AIDS virus is also called
    a. HAV
    b. LAV
    c. IMV
    d. CMV
15. Name two opportunistic diseases that commonly affect the AIDS patient.
16. The period when neither antigens nor antibodies are detected in the serum of a patient affected with the AIDS virus is called a/an
    a. inactive stage
    b. nonactive stage
    c. window phase
    d. door phase
17. Cytomegalovirus is a
    a. herpesvirus
    b. hepadnavirus
    c. togavirus
    d. retrovirus

FURTHER ACTIVITIES

Invite a speaker from the local AIDS network to speak on AIDS or an individual with AIDS who addresses the subject of living with AIDS.

Show films on AIDS and hepatitis. Suggestions include films dealing with the history of AIDS (*And The Band Played On*) or the consequences of living with AIDS (*Philadelphia*).

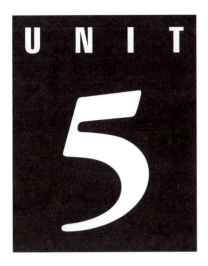

UNIT 5

Febrile Diseases

After studying this unit, the student should know the following objectives:

- Discuss the principle of the C-reactive protein (CPR) test.

- Discuss causes of the rise of acute-phase protein.

- Discuss diseases caused by *Streptococcus pyogenes.*

- Discuss the exoenzymes produced by *Streptococcus pyogenes.*

- Explain the reason for keeping the blood specimen warm when it is drawn for a cold agglutinin test.

- Discuss clinical symptoms of mycoplasma pneumonia

- Discuss the diseases tested for in the febrile antigen slide test.

GLOSSARY

Antistreptolysin O, (ASO): An antibody produced in response to *Streptococcus pyogenes.*

Brucella: Causative agent of undulant fever.

C-reactive protein (CRP): Acute-phase protein produced in response to inflammation.

Cross reaction: Antibody reaction of two different strains of organisms reacting against the same antigen.

ESR: Abbreviation for erythrocyte sedimentation rate.

Exoenzyme: An enzyme that does not function with the cell it was created in.

Extracellular: Outside of the cell

Febrile antigen: A foreign protein that will cause the body to produce a fever.

Malignant: Harmful.

Nephelometry: Measurement of the turbidity in a fluid.

Nonpathogen: Organism that does not cause disease.

Pathogen: Organism that causes disease.

Proteus: Gram-negative organism found in the intestine.

Rheumatoid arthritis (RA): A chronic inflammatory disease in which the joints become inflamed, painful, and swollen.

Rickettsia: A genus of organisms intermediate between viruses and bacteria.

Salmonella: Gram-negative enteric organism commonly found in the small intestine.

Salmonella typhi: Causative agent of typhoid fever

Systemic lupus erythematosus (SLE): A chronic inflammatory disease first affecting the bones, muscles, and eventually all parts of the body.

Turbidimetry: Estimation of the turbidity (muddiness or cloudiness) of a liquid.

INTRODUCTION

Febrile diseases are those diseases caused by microorganisms that produce an elevated temperature in the patient.

Microorganisms have been on earth in great numbers since the world began. Most of the time the human body has a strong defense against these organisms. As discussed in Unit 1, intact skin is one of the best defenses the body has against bacteria and other organisms.

Many microbes, such as *Staphylococcus epidermidis,* are normally on our skin and cause no harm. The type of microorganism that is not harmful to the body is called a **nonpathogen.** Microorganisms that are harmful to the body are called **pathogens.**

The serology department performs tests to determine if the body has been invaded not only by bacteria but also by microorganisms named ***rickettsia.*** One test procedure is a nonspecific type of test for acute-phase protein. Other tests determine the presence or absence of antibodies to bacterial or rickettsial invasion.

ACUTE-PHASE PROTEIN, OR C-REACTIVE PROTEIN*

The **C-reactive protein (CRP)** is synthesized in the liver and has a half-life of 20 to 30 hours.

The CRP belongs to the so-called acute-phase proteins whose serum concentration increases during the course of a general, nonspecific response to infectious and inflammatory processes, cellular necrosis, and malignant neoplasias. The CRP contributes to nonspecific defense by complement activation and acceleration of phagocytosis.

Although the CRP concentration is generally less than 5 mg/L in the serum of healthy adults, in a number of disease states these values are often exceeded within four to eight hours after an acute event and reach levels of about 20 to 500 mg/L. Because an elevated CRP level is always associated with pathological changes, determination of CRP is a more sensitive and reliable indicator of inflammatory processes than either the erythrocyte sedimentation rate **(ESR)** or the leukocyte count. Increases in the serum CRP concentration occur faster than those of the ESR, and when the condition subsides, CRP levels fall very quickly, reaching normal levels several days before the ESR normalizes.

Determination of CRP is particularly advisable in the following situations:

1. Screening for inflammatory and necrotic processes.
2. Diagnosis and monitoring of treatment of infections and inflammatory processes such as neonatal septicemia, meningitis, pneumonia, pyelonephritis, postoperative complications, and **malignant** conditions (especially in combination with other acute-phase proteins and tumor markers).

*The following information on the RapiTek CRP procedure was obtained from Behring Diagnostics, Inc., and is used with their permission.

3. Assessment of the clinical picture in inflammatory conditions such as those of the rheumatic type or during acute episodes or intermittent infections.
4. Differential diagnosis of inflammatory conditions such as **systemic lupus erythematosus (SLE), rheumatoid arthritis (RA)** or other arthritic diseases, Crohn's disease (colitis ulcerosa), and acute cystitis (pyelonephritis).

The CRP can be determined by capillary precipitation, Ouchterlony double diffusion, radial immunodiffusion, and nephelometry.

RAPITEX CRP TEST

RapiTex CRP is a simple latex agglutination procedure that can be performed rapidly. Qualitative and semiquantitative results are available, but for precise quantitation, radial immunodiffusion, **nephelometry,** or **turbidimetry** is recommended.

Principles. The test is based on immunological reaction between CRP antibodies to CRP bound to latex particles. Elevated CRP concentrations (> 6 mg/L) lead to visible agglutination of the latex particles.

EXERCISE   **19**   QUALITATIVE CRP METHOD

Following the manufacturer's instructions, have the students perform a test on serum for CRP.

1. Warm the CRP kit to room temperature.
2. Read the manufacturer's instructions
3. Pipette 40 μl of undiluted patient sample onto separate fields on the slide. Place one drop of the positive and one drop of the negative control serum on separate fields of the test slide.
4. Place one drop (approximately 40 μl) of the Absorption Solution for RapiTex CRP adjacent to each sample.
5. Gently mix the contents of the RapiTex reagent bottle (including contents of dropper). Fill dropper with well-mixed suspension and place one drop next to the sample of Absorption Solution drop on each field of the test slide. Thoroughly mix the three drops in each field with a stirring rod. Use a clean stirring rod for each section of the slide.
6. Rotate the slide through several planes. After two minutes, examine for agglutination.

EXERCISE ▪ 20 ▪ SEMIQUANTITATIVE CRP METHOD

Have the students follow the manufacturer's directions to perform a semiquantitative CRP.

1. Prepare dilutions of the patient's serum with isotonic saline solution for this test method, according to the following scheme: receiving 0.5 ml/tube (Figure 5.1).
2. Pipette 40 μml of the patient's diluted serum into separate fields on the slide. Place one drop of the positive and one drop of the negative control serum in a separate field on the slide.
3. Place one drop (approximately 40 μl) of the Absorption Solution adjacent to each sample.
4. Gently mix the contents of the reagent bottle and place one drop next to the sample of Adsorption Solution on the test slide.
5. Thoroughly mix the three drops in each field using a clean a stirring rod for each field.
6. Continuously rotate the slide through several planes. After two minutes, examine for agglutination.

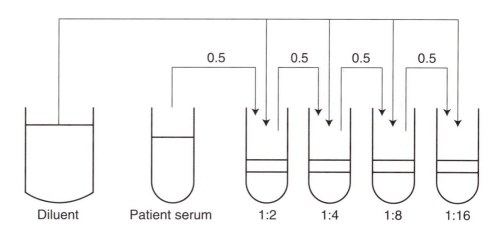

fig. 5.1. CRP dilution

Specimens. Fresh serum or plasma collected using heparin or ethylenediaminetetraacetic acid (EDTA) samples are suitable. Samples can be stored frozen ($\leq -25°C$) up to 3 months if they are frozen within 24 hours of collection and are not repeatedly thawed and refrozen.

Serum samples must have clotted completely and contain no particulate matter or any traces of fibrin after centrifugation. Very lipemic samples or samples that become turbid after thawing should be clarified by centrifugation (10 minutes at $15,000 \times G$) before assay.

Table 5.1. Semiquantitative Evaluation of CRP

Dilution Agglutinating	CRP Concentration (approx. mg/L)
	± 20%
1:2	≥ 12%
1:4	≥ 24%
1:8	≥ 48%
1:16	≥ 96%

Chart used with permission by Behringwerke AG/Behring Diagnostics, Inc., Somerville, N.J.

Qualitative CRP Results. Distinct agglutination identifies a CRP concen-tration greater than 6 mg/L in the sample; samples that do not react with RapiTex CRP contain CRP concentrations less than 6 mg/L.

Internal Quality Control. Controls must be included in each test series. Positive CRP Control Serum must show distinct agglutination, whereas the negative Control Serum must not react when tested.

Semiquantitative CRP Results. The highest sample dilution that still shows distinct agglutination is evaluated. The CRP content of the patient sample is taken from Table 5.1.

Limitations and Interferences. Reading the tests after more than two minutes can lead to false-positive results. Lipemic sera and plasma can also cause nonspecific reactions.

The strength of agglutination is not indicative of the CRP concentration. In the qualitative test, weak reactions may occur with markedly elevated concentrations. Agglutination reactions are weaker between 300 and 400 mg/L than at lower concentrations, but no false negatives were found up to 400 mg/L. When CRP concentrations greater than 400 mg/L are expected, the sample should be tested diluted. Rheumatoid factors (RFs) can cause false-positive results in latex agglutination tests. The Absorption Solution for RapiTex CRP minimizes such interference of RF concentrations up to approximately 1,200 IU/ml. If the RF concentration of a sample exceeds 1,200 IU/ml, the sample should be evaluated by a different test method (e.g., radial immunodiffusion or nephelometry).

Reference Intervals. In healthy adults, the serum CRP concentrations are less than 5 mg/L. Because CRP is an unspecific indicator for various disease processes, reference ranges are subject to many influence parameters that may differ for every investigated group. Every laboratory should establish the relevant upper limit of the reference range itself.

STREPTOCOCCUS PYOGENES

Streptococcus pyogenes is a gram-positive coccus that causes human infections. This organism can be divided into groups A, B, C, and G. The β-Hemolytic *Streptococcus,* Lancefield Group A, receives more attention than the other groups. This organism causes pharyngitis and upper respiratory tract infections, and if not treated adequately or left untreated, it can cause the infected person to develop rheumatic fever, which can cause heart damage and glomerulonephritis (damage to glomerulus in the kidney).

Tests have been developed to detect the antibodies resulting from *S. pyogenes* infections. These tests use **extracellular** products produced in response to the bacteria. These products are: (1) **antistreptolysin O (ASO);** (2) antihyaluronidase (AH), which breaks down hyaluronic acid found in human connective tissue; (3) antistreptokinase (ASK), an enzyme that dissolves clots; (4) antideoxyriboneuclease (ADN-B), which degrades deoxyribonucleic acid; and (5) antinicotinamide adenine dinucleotidase (ANAD), which elicits antibody response (e.g., esterase or amylase).

The ASO is a globulin that can combine with and fix streptolysin O, neutralizing it in vitro and rendering it incapable of lysing red blood cells.

One of the first serological tests devised was the ASO titer, a neutralization test. This procedure uses diluted patient serum plus streptolysin O reagent and washed human red blood cells (blood group O). Controls are set up with two tests, one a red blood cell control and the second a streptolysin control. These dilutions are incubated at 37°C and read for tubes showing no hemolysis. This procedure is reported in Todd units. Titers greater than 166 Todd units are diagnostically significant.

As with other serological tests, one serum specimen test is not enough on which to base a diagnosis. A blood specimen should be drawn again in 14 days and a second test performed. If the titer rises, it is suggestive of an increase in infections. A declining titer indicates recovery.

A second test method for ASO is a latex agglutination test. The ASO product (antigen) is fixed on the surface of latex particles. These latex particles are mixed

E X E R C I S E **21** **ASO AND RELATED EXOENZYME TESTING**

Have the students perform a test procedure for ASO and related **exoenzymes.**

1. Place the kit at room temperature to warm.
2. Read the manufacturer's instructions.
3. Dilute the patient serum 1:100 with isotonic saline solution (9.9 ml of saline solution + 0.1 ml of serum)
4. Place 0.05 ml of diluted sample on the test slide.
5. Place one drop of positive control and one drop of negative control in the marked areas of the test slide.
6. Add one drop of the reagent provided in the kit to each of the marked areas of the test slide.
7. With a clean stirring rod, mix each of the serums and cells in the marked areas of the slide.
8. Rock the slide back and forth gently for 2 minutes. Place the slide on a flat surface and observe for agglutination within 10 seconds.
9. Agglutination is a positive test result and indicates that the test must be titered.
10. Discuss the test principle stated by the manufacturer of the test kit.

with the patient's diluted serum on a slide and rotated. If the latex particles agglutinate, the test result is positive. If there is no agglutination, the test result is negative. If the qualitative test result is positive, it can be quantitated to determine the amount of ASO present.

A third test method for ASO uses sheep red blood cells to which *Streptococcus* Group A extracellular antigens have been fixed. The patient's diluted serum is reacted with the sheep cells on a slide. If streptococcal antibodies are present, the red blood cells will agglutinate. This type of a procedure is a hemagglutination test. The antibody, if present, can be quantitated. This test will detect the five antibodies that can be produced against *S. pyogenes;* however, the test does not differentiate any one of the antibodies from the others.

COLD AGGLUTININS

Cold agglutinins are found in low titer in almost all human serum. If the patient is infected with *Mycoplasma pneumoniae,* the cold agglutinin titer will rise significantly. The disease mycoplasma pneumonia occurs usually in young adults. The patient complaints are chills, fever, headache, sore throat, gastrointestinal symptoms, and a cough. These symptoms are the same as symptoms of other disease processes. If the patient has a chest radiograph, the radiograph will be positive for pneumonia.

Specimen Collection. Unlike other serological procedures, the blood specimen for cold agglutinins must be handled differently after collection.

The blood specimen for this test is a clotted specimen, although there is a procedure for cold agglutinin titers that uses blood collected in EDTA, which also gives the same results.

When the blood specimen is drawn, it must be kept warm until the serum is removed from the cells. Once the serum has been removed, it can be refrigerated if the test procedure will be delayed. However, the serum must be returned to room temperature before the test procedure is set up.

The serum of patients with mycoplasma pneumonia will agglutinate red blood cells in the cold at 4°C to 6°C but not at 37°C. The antibody produced by this organism is termed a cold-reacting antibody.

These cold-reacting antibodies are nonspecific and are found in other diseases, such as Raynaud's syndrome and cirrhosis.

Cold agglutinins in mycoplasma pneumonia appear during the first week of the disease. The titer will rise from day 8 to day 25 and then begin to decline.

The test procedure for cold antibodies produced in response to mycoplasma pneumonia is a hemagglutination test.

The patient's serum is diluted twofold in isotonic saline solution. A 1% cell suspension of human blood group O cells is added to the diluted saline and serum mixture. The patient's red blood cells can be used in place of other human blood group O cells.

The tubes are refrigerated for 1 hour at 4°C. At the end of the hour, the tubes are gently shaken and examined for agglutination of the red blood cells. A notation of the highest dilution that agglutinated the cells is made. The titer will be the highest dilution of the serum that agglutinated the cells after refrigeration. The tubes are then incubated at 37°C for 30 minutes. After incubation the tubes are gently shaken to determine if the agglutination has dispersed.

E X E R C I S E   22   COLD AGGLUTININ TITER

Have the students perform a cold agglutinin titer.

1. Prepare the serum specimen. Warm to room temperature.
2. Assemble tubes, pipettes, saline solution, and tube racks.
3. Wash the appropriate red blood cells and prepare a 1% saline cell suspension.
4. Prepare a twofold serial dilution of the serum.
5. Add appropriate amount of red blood cells to the tubes.
6. Refrigerate for one hour and read the tubes for agglutination. *Do not centrifuge the tubes*.
7. Incubate the agglutinated tubes at 37°C for 30 minutes.
8. Read the tubes for lack of agglutination.
9. Record the highest dilution that had agglutination after refrigeration.
10. Discuss the principle of the test procedure.

If the agglutination did not disperse after 37°C incubation, it is an indication that something other than cold antibodies are present in the serum or plasma.

Normal titers for this test are less than 1:64 dilution. Any titer greater than 1:64 is abnormal.

Unlike other serological procedures, the height of the titer of cold agglutinins indicates the severity of the disease.

FEBRILE ANTIGENS*

Febrile antigen is a term that refers to bacterial suspensions representative of a number of species of microorganisms pathogenic to humans that are accompanied by a fever in the host. There are a number of such organisms, the most prominent include the genera **Salmonella, Brucella,** *Francisella (Pasteurella), Leptospira,* and some members of the genus *Rickettsia*.

One test quantitatively measures the agglutinins in the sera of patients with typhoid fever. This test also includes *Salmonella* species other than *Salmonella typhi* by use of a variety of *Salmonella* O and H antigens. This test is called the Widal test.

Another set of antigens are used to test for agglutinins to the causative agent of typhus fever, *Rickettsia prowazekii,* and strains of *Proteus vulgaris.* The strains of **Proteus** are Ox19, OX2, and OXK. This test is called the Weil-Felix test.

Some antibodies produced by one organism may demonstrate a **cross reaction** with antibodies produced by another organism. *R. prowazekii* and certain strains of *P. vulgaris* demonstrate this cross reaction.

*The following information about the Bacto-Febrile Antigen Set is reproduced with permission from Difco Laboratories, Detroit.

A test procedure for the detection of the antibodies produced in typhoid fever and typhus fever is available.

This rapid slide test, including the Widal and Weil-Felix reactions, usually employs six or more antigens from bacteria commonly causing fever in the host. A *Proteus* OX19 suspension is used to detect rickettsial antibodies. Varying amounts of the sera to be tested are distributed to the corresponding square of a previously marked glass slide. A febrile antigen is added and mixed with the sera. Positive or negative results are read one minute after mixing.

The rapid slide test is the most widely used procedure employing febrile antigens because of the simplicity with which the results may be reported (Figure 5.2). Negative reactions with this test can usually be reported as such if all five serum dilutions have been used. Even though the slide test is not quantitative, it is necessary to run the series of dilutions in order (one to six tubes) to detect agglutinin content of a serum that might be overlooked in the case of a "prozone reaction." This often occurs in the sera containing *Brucella* agglutinins and to a lesser extent typhoid agglutinins where higher concentrations of the serum may yield negative results but, when the serum is diluted, the results may be positive.

The macroscopic tube test should be used to confirm the presence of antibodies demonstrated by the slide technique and to quantitate their titer in suspected sera (Figure 5.3). In this test the patients's serum is serially diluted in test tubes, a constant amount of the appropriate dilution of a febrile antigen is added each tube, the resultant mixture is incubated according to directions, and the agglutination pattern is read and recorded.

Agglutination

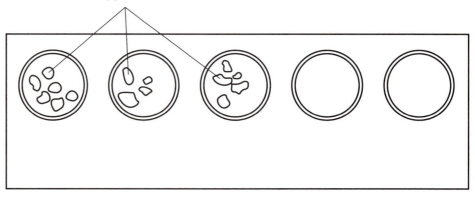

fig. 5.2. Febrile antigen slide test

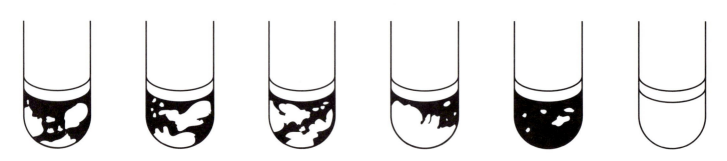

fig. 5.3. Febrile antigen tube test

Record results as follows:

4+ Complete agglutination

3+ Approximately 75% of the cells are clumped

2+ Approximately 50% of the cells are clumped

1+ Approximately 25% of the cells are clumped

+ Trace agglutination

− No agglutination

The titer of the serum is recorded as that dilution of the specimen in which at least 2+ (50% agglutination) occurs (Table 5.2).

Table 5.2. Sample Calculations Rapid Slide Test

Serum (ml)	Corrected Dilution	Spec 1	Spec 2	Spec 3
0.08	1:20	3+	4+	4+
0.04	1:40	2+	4+	3+
0.02	1:80	1+	3+	2+
0.01	1:160	−	3+	+
0.005	1:320	−	1+	−
Serum titer		1:40	1:160	1:80

E X E R C I S E　23　**FEBRILE ANTIGEN TUBE TEST**

Have the students perform a febrile antigen test.

1. Assemble pipettes and slides needed for the test.
2. Read the manufacturer's instructions.
3. Pipette 0.08, 0.04, 0.02, 0.01, and 0.005 ml of serum into a row of squares on the ruled glass plate using a 0.2-ml serological pipette.
4. Place a drop of the appropriate antigen for the slide test on each drop of serum. Note: Shake the antigen well before using.
5. Mix each serum-antigen composite with an applicator stick starting with the 0.005-ml serum dilution and work toward the 0.08-ml dilution.
6. Hold the glass plate in both hands and gently "rotate" it 15 to 20 times. Observe the agglutination within 1 minute over a suitable light source.
7. The final dilutions are 1:20, 1:40, 1:80, 1:160, and 1:320, respectively.
8. Adhere strictly to the time limitations of the test.

CALIBRATION AND QUALITY CONTROL

Both positive and negative controls are diluted in the same proportion as the patient's serum and processed in exactly the same manner after the procedure just discussed for the rapid slide test or the macroscopic tube test.

An antigen is considered to be satisfactory if it does not clump with the negative control and it reacts to a titer of 1:80 or more with the positive control.

INTERPRETATION

Table 5.3 lists febrile antigens and their titers for a variety of pathologies.

1. Although the febrile antigens are useful for screening purposes, the technique should not be a complete substitute for the conventional isolation and serological identification of the etiological agent.
2. The rapid slide test should be used for screening only. Any positive results in the slide procedure should be confirmed by the tube test.
3. For greater proficiency in test interpretation, always include a positive and negative serum control in each test protocol.
4. Serum from cases of typhoid fever often agglutinate with *Salmonella* O antigen Group B (paratyphoid B) but rarely with group A antigen.
5. Significant titers may be obtained in specimens immunized with tetanus antitoxin (TAT) and typhoid vaccines.
6. Nonspecific agglutination has been noted with *Salmonella* O antigen Group D in sera from patients with influenza.
7. Reciprocal cross reactions with *Tularensis* and *Brucella* agglutinins and antigens have been reported.
8. The *Brucella* antigen may cross react with persons immunized with cholera vaccine.
9. Some normal material sera may possess a titer to the *Proteus* antigen.

Table 5.3. Febrile Antigens and Titers

Antigen	Pathology	Time of Maximum titer	Significant Titer
B. Abortus	Brucellosis	3–5 weeks	1:80 (≥ 1:160 indicative)
Proteus OX 19	Rocky Mountain spotted fever	2–3 weeks	1:160–1:320
Proteus OX 19	Typhus	2–3 weeks	1:160
Salmonella H antigen d (typhoid H)	Typhoid	4–5 weeks	1:80
Salmonella O antigen D (typhoid O)	Typhoid fever	3–5 weeks	1:80 *
Salmonella H antigen a (paratyphoid A)	Paratyphoid fever	3–5 weeks	1:80 *
Salmonella H antigen b (paratyphoid B)	Paratyphoid fever	3–5 weeks	1:80 *

* Significant in nonvaccinated individuals.

10. Sera from narcotic addicts appear to contain broad nonspecific activity to the febrile antigen.
11. Sera from patients with chronic active liver disease may demonstrate high agglutinin titers.
12. Report the serum titer as the reciprocal of the highest dilution showing a 2+ reaction.
13. In some cases of brucellosis, sera may demonstrate a prozone (the inability of an antigen to react in higher serum concentrations). All five serum dilutions should be run in the rapid slide test rather than just one dilution to eliminate the possibility of missing positive reactions due to prozone.

SUMMARY

Microorganisms such as bacteria are normally found on the skin *(S. epidermidis)* and in the intestinal tract *(Escherichia coli),* and cause no harm to the body if they do not enter the body through a break in the skin or a break in the intestinal lining. (A break in the intestinal lining can be caused by ulceration or surgery.) These organisms are called nonpathogens. If these organisms enter the bloodstream, they can cause disease processes. Then they are called pathogens.

The body will produce acute-phase protein in large amounts when there is an infection or inflammation in the body. This acute-phase protein is CRP. A rise in CRP can be detected by a qualitative and a semiquantitative latex agglutination procedure.

S. pyogenes is gram-positive cocci that can produce toxins harmful to the patient; some of the disease processes caused by *S. pyogenes* are pharyngitis, glomerulonephritis, and rheumatic fever. The *S. pyogenes* cocci belongs to Lancefield Group A.

Extracellular products to *S. pyogenes* infections are ASO, AH, ASK, ADN-B, and ANAD.

The first test procedure devised was the antistreptolysin O titer, which is a neutralization test.

A second test method to determine the amount of antistreptolysin in the serum is a latex agglutination method. A third test method is a hemagglutination method using sheep erythrocytes (red blood cells). This third method detects the five exoenzymes produced in the serum in response to *S. pyogenes*.

Mycoplasma pneumonia is a bacterial infection to which the body will produce antibodies that react in the cold (4°C to 6°C).

The test procedure for detection of these cold antibodies utilizes the patient's serum and the patient's red blood cells or the patient's serum and any human blood group O cell. This procedure is a hemagglutination test.

The Widal test using *Salmonella* H and O antigens is used for detecting typhoid fever and paratyphoid fever.

The Weil-Felix test uses a strain of the bacteria *Proteus* as the antigen to detect antibodies present in typhus and Rocky Mountain spotted fever.

The Widal and Weil-Felix tests are agglutination tests performed as a rapid slide test. If the tests are positive for any of the antibodies formed, the test can then be performed as a tube test titer.

REVIEW QUESTIONS

1. CRP is synthesized in the
   a. kidney
   b. liver
   c. pancreas
   d. gallbladder

2. CRP can be determined by all of the following *except*
   a. radioimmunoassay
   b. radial immunodiffusion
   c. nephelometry
   d. double diffusion

3. Internal quality control procedures consist of
   a. positive controls
   b. negative controls
   c. a only
   d. both a and b

4. Most normal healthy adult serum contains CRP concentrations
   a. < 2 mg/L
   b. < 5 mg/L
   c. > 5 mg/L
   d. > 7 mg/L

5. The sample for CRP testing should be evaluated by a different method if the rheumatoid factor in serum is greater than what number?
   a. 500 IU/ml
   b. 700 IU/ml
   c. 900 IU/ml
   d. 1,200 IU/ml

6. *Streptococcus pyogenes* is a
   a. gram-negative coccus
   b. gram-positive coccus
   c. gram-negative bacillus
   d. gram-positive bacillus

7. β-Hemolytic *S. pyogenes* is of the Lancefield Group
   a. G
   b. B
   c. A
   d. C

8. The ASO titer is reported in
   a. Todd units
   b. International units
   c. mg%
   d. g/dl

9. *S. pyogenes* infections produce how many exotoxins in the serum?
    a. 2
    b. 3
    c. 5
    d. 7
10. In the ASO titer procedure the tubes are read for
    a. hemolysis
    b. no hemolysis
    c. agglutination
    d. precipitation
11. One test method for determining the presence of antibodies to *S. pyogenes* used what type of erythrocytes in the procedure?
    a. horse
    b. goat
    c. sheep
    d. human
12. One of the causative agents that produce an elevation of cold-reacting antibody is
    a. *S. pyogenes*
    b. *S. typhi*
    c. *P. vulgaris*
    d. *Mycoplasma pneumoniae*
13. What is the name of the test procedure for cold agglutinins?
    a. hemagglutination
    b. neutralization
    c. precipitation
    d. hemolysin
14. The ASO titer is what type of test?
    a. hemagglutination
    b. neutralization
    c. precipitation
    d. hemolysin
15. The dilution for a cold agglutinin titer is
    a. twofold
    b. threefold
    c. fourfold
    d. none
16. The cells used in the cold agglutinin titer are
    a. horse
    b. human
    c. sheep
    d. goat
17. Febrile refers to
    a. chill
    b. fever
    c. chills and fever
    d. none of the above

18. The rapid slide test for febrile agglutinins must be titered to detect
    a. prozone reactions
    b. postzone reactions
    c. both a and b
    d. neither a nor b

19. *S. typhi* is the causative agent of
    a. typhoid fever
    b. scrub typhus
    c. brucellosis
    d. tularemia

20. The antigens used in the Widal test are
    a. *Salmonella* O
    b. *Salmonella* H
    c. *S. typhi*
    d. all of the above

21. The antigens used in the Weil-Felix test are
    a. *Salmonella* O
    b. *Salmonella* H
    c. *S. typhi*
    d. *Proteus*

FURTHER ACTIVITIES

Have the students prepare a case study that includes clinical symptoms and laboratory findings for each of the disease processes in this unit.

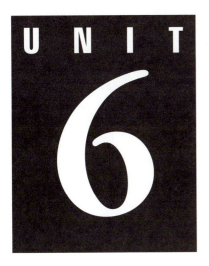

Autoimmune Diseases

LEARNING OBJECTIVES

After studying this unit, the student should be able to:

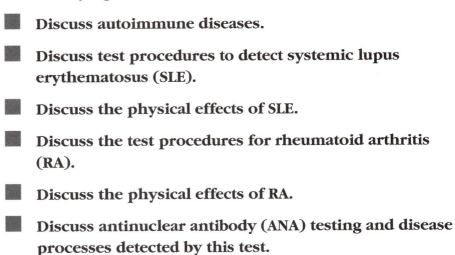

- Discuss autoimmune diseases.

- Discuss test procedures to detect systemic lupus erythematosus (SLE).

- Discuss the physical effects of SLE.

- Discuss the test procedures for rheumatoid arthritis (RA).

- Discuss the physical effects of RA.

- Discuss antinuclear antibody (ANA) testing and disease processes detected by this test.

GLOSSARY

Antinuclear antibody (ANA): Antibody directed against the nucleus of test cells.

Anemia: Lack of red blood cells in the circulatory system.

Autoimmune hemolytic anemia: Destruction of red blood cells by the body.

Hep-2 cells: Liver cells used in ANA testing.

Hypochromic: Decreased color. Used to describe red blood cells without the normal amount of hemoglobin.

Microcytic: Adjective used to describe small red blood cells (microcytes).

Nephritis: Inflamation of the nephrons in the kidneys.

Normochromic: Possessing normal color.

Normocytic: Having normal size.

Pernicious anemia: Severe form of blood disease.

Rheumatoid arthritis (RA): A disease affecting the joints of the body.

Scleroderma: A chronic disease that causes the skin to harden.

Sjögren's syndrome: Appears in postmenopausal women.

Systemic lupus erythematosus (SLE): Chronic inflammatory disease of connective tissue.

INTRODUCTION

In autoimmune diseases, the human body loses its ability to distinguish between self and non-self. The immune system will build antibodies against its own tissue, which then becomes the antigen.

There are many types of autoimmune diseases, such as **autoimmune hemolytic anemia, pernicious anemia,** and multiple sclerosis.

This unit will address two of the most common auto-immune diseases and the serological test procedures to detect the antibodies in the serum.

SYSTEMIC LUPUS ERYTHEMATOSUS

There is no known cause of **systemic lupus erythematosus (SLE).** The disease could be the result of a primary defect in the regulation of the immune system; however, SLE can also be drug related. Certain drugs, such as prednisone, administered to the patient will give a false-positive serum test result for SLE. The word lupus comes from the Latin word for wolf.

More women than men have SLE. The SLE symptoms will worsen during pregnancy.

CLINICAL SYMPTOMS

Patients with SLE have clinical symptoms featuring a skin rash, usually on the face across the nose and cheeks. The rash often appears in the shape of a butterfly. This rash is appropriately called a butterfly rash. Other symptoms include arthritis and **nephritis.**

LABORATORY TESTING

Patients have a mild to moderate **anemia** of the **normocytic-normochromic** variety. Some patients will have autoimmune hemolytic anemia due to a positive direct antihuman globulin test result. A direct antihuman globulin test is performed on patient's erythrocytes (red blood cells) to detect antibodies or complement that may have attached in the patient's body and are destroying the red blood cells. Both antibodies and complement can cause the cell to hemolyze. About half of the patients will have leukopenia (decreased white blood cell count).

Patients with SLE develop abnormal plasma proteins or autoantibodies. The SLE patient serum will give a false positive test result for **rheumatoid arthritis (RA)** and also for syphilis.

RHEUMATOID ARTHRITIS

Rheumatoid arthritis (RA) is a chronic disease that affects the joints with inflammation, stiffness, and soreness. Most individuals affected with RA have a gradual onset of the disease, but usually all of the joints in the body will be affected. As the disease progresses, other organs in the body (e.g., lungs and heart) can develop an inflammatory condition.

Rheumatoid arthritis affects men, women, and children. There is a tendency for more females than males to be affected by the disease.

Laboratory findings in patients with RA may have a mild anemia, which is normocytic and normochromic. In a low percentage of patients the anemia is microcytic and **hypochromic.** The leukocyte count may be slightly elevated. The C-reactive protein (CRP) level and erythrocyte sedimentation rate (ESR) will be elevated, indicating an inflammatory process in the body.

The immunoglobulins associated with rheumatoid factor are IgG, IgM, and IgA. These antibodies have a specificity for altered IgG.

Does the altered IgG cause the inflammatory condition? Or is RA an inflammatory response against the inflammatory condition? These questions remain unanswered.

The most important rheumatoid factor in laboratory testing is the IgM macroglobulin. In vivo the altered IgG combines with rheumatoid factor and complement. The IgM macroglobulin is produced by plasma cells of the B-cell origin. Because IgM can be produced against other disease processes or organisms, the level of IgM can be elevated and not be the IgM macroglobulin produced in response to RA.

The tests for rheumatoid factor rely on the agglutinating properties of the IgM antibody in the serum.

Human or rabbit IgG is bound to a carrier particle, usually a latex particle or, in some test methods, a charcoal particle. If IgM antibody to RA is in the serum, the carrier particles will agglutinate.

EXERCISE 24 LATEX SLIDE TEST FOR RHEUMATOID FACTOR

Have the students assemble the materials needed for the test procedure.

1. Warm the kit to room temperature.
2. Read the manufacturer's instructions.
3. Prepare a 1:20 dilution of the patient's serum in buffer solution provided in the kit. 0.1 ml of serum + 1.9 ml of buffer.
4. Place 0.05 ml of the serum-cell mixture on the slide.
5. Mix the latex reagent thoroughly and add one drop to the serum-cell mixture on the slide.
6. Mix well with a stirring rod.
7. Rotate the slide by hand for two minutes.
8. Read the slide macroscopically for agglutination.
9. Positive and negative controls must be performed with the procedure.
10. Results:
    Agglutination = positive test result
    No agglutination = negative test result

The latex agglutination test methods are performed on a slide. If the test result is positive, it can then be titered in tubes. If the qualitative test is positive, perform a quantitative test procedure.

Another type of test for RA is an adaption of the RPR card test for syphilis. In this procedure, charcoal particles are the carrier of the IgG molecule. The test is performed like the RPR card test for syphilis.

ANTINUCLEAR ANTIBODY TESTING

Antinuclear antibody (ANA) testing is performed to detect antibodies in the serum (circulating antibodies) to nuclear antigens. The antibodies are directed against the nucleus of the test cells being used, hence the name antinuclear.

The ANA testing will detect SLE, RA, connective tissue diseases, **scleroderma,** and **Sjögren's syndrome.**

FLUORESCENT ANTINUCLEAR ANTIBODY TESTING (FANA)

One type of test procedure used to detect nuclear antibodies to nuclear antigens is a fluorescent (FANA) test. The test involves reacting tissue cells on a slide with the patient's serum to which a tagged antibody against γ-globulin is added. The

EXERCISE 25 LATEX QUANTITATIVE TEST FOR RHEUMATOID ARTHRITIS

1. Label 10 12 × 75 mm tubes numbers 1 to 10.
2. Pipette 1.9 ml of buffer into tube number 1.
3. Pipette 1.0 ml of buffer into tubes number 2 through 10.
4. Pipette 0.1 ml of the patient's serum into tube number 1. Mix and transfer 1.0 ml of the mixture to tube number 2.
5. Continue to transfer 1.0 ml from tube number 2 to tube number 9. Discard 1.0 ml from tube number 9.
6. *Do not add the patient's diluted serum to tube number 10. This is a negative control tube.*
7. Place one drop of thoroughly mixed latex antigen into tubes number 1 through 10.
8. Incubate all tubes at 37°C for 15 minutes.
9. At the end of the incubation period, centrifuge all tubes on low speed for appropriate time.
10. Gently shake the tubes to resuspend the antigen. Examine each tube macroscopically for agglutination. Tube number 10 should have no agglutination.
11. The titer is the last tube with agglutination. Dilutions are 1:20, 1:40, 1:80, 1:160, and so on.

tagged antibody is a fluorescein polyvalent antihuman globulin. The tissue cells on the slide are usually rat liver cells.

The slides are examined with a fluorescence microscope to detect cells on the slide that fluoresce and to determine the pattern of fluorescence. The cells are graded from 0 to 4. Positive and negative controls are performed with the test. The pattern detected will be an indication of the type of disease condition of the patient. The patterns are rim, solid, speckled, nucleolar, and anticentromere.

CHEMICAL ANTINUCLEAR ANTIBODY TESTS

These procedures are enzyme techniques using horseradish peroxidase–bound antihuman globulin. In the procedure diluted human serum is incubated with rat liver cells **(Hep-2 cells)** fixed on a slide. After incubation, the slide is reacted with the horseradish peroxidase bound with antihuman globulin. The test is read microscopically by brightfield microscope looking for pattern reactions of the cells on the slide. The patterns are rim (seen in SLE), homogenous (seen in SLE and RA), nucleolar (seen in scleroderma and Sjögren's syndrome), speckled (detecting smooth muscle antigen), and anticentromere (ANAs against centromere antigen, suggestive of systemic sclerosis).

Positive and negative controls must be performed with the test procedure. Positive controls are available for all of the patterns.

ANAs can also be detected by solid-phase fluorescent immunoassay. Liver (Hep-2) cells are fixed to the test strips used in the test procedure. This test is a quantitative test, and the pattern can be determined by use of a fluorescence microscope.

SUMMARY

In autoimmune diseases, the human body loses its ability to differentiate between self and non-self and builds antibodies against its own tissue. The body's tissue acts as the antigen.

The most common autoimmune diseases are SLE and RA. Both conditions have similar clinical manifestations and some similarities in laboratory procedure reactions.

The SLE disease can give a false-positive reaction for RA and syphilis. The disease process causes a skin rash across the cheeks, arthritis, and nephritis.

The test procedures used for detection of SLE are FANA tests, chemical procedures utilizing enzymes, and solid-phase immunofluorescence.

RA is an autoimmune disease affecting joints and organs. It is more common in females than males.

Rheumatoid factor is an altered IgG immunoglobulin that reacts with complement in the plasma in vivo.

Several laboratory test procedures detect the presence of rheumatoid factors in the serum. The most commonly used procedure uses IgG antibody bound to latex particles to detect the IgM macroglobulin in the serum of patients with RA. This method can be quantitated.

Other test procedures use charcoal particles with bound IgG adapted to the principles of the rapid plasma reagin (RPR) serological card test for syphilis (see Unit 3).

Testing for ANA can be performed using chemical slide procedures and solid-phase immunofluorescence.

REVIEW QUESTIONS

1. Clinical symptoms of SLE and RA are similar.
   a. true
   b. false

2. A butterfly rash is found in
   a. lupus
   b. RA
   c. pernicious anemia
   d. none of the above

3. RA affects
   a. males
   b. females
   c. children
   d. all of the above

4. SLE and RA can cause inflammation of the joints.
   a. true
   b. false

5. In autoimmune diseases, antibody and complement can cause the hemolysis of red blood cells.
   a. true
   b. false

6. Leukopenia is a/an
   a. increase in red blood cells
   b. decrease in red blood cells
   c. increase in white blood cells
   d. decrease in white blood cells

7. The macroglobulin produced in RA is
   a. IgA
   b. IgG
   c. IgM
   d. IgD

8. The immunoglobulin used to coat carrier particles for RA testing is
   a. IgA
   b. IgG
   c. IgM
   d. IgD

9. A latex test for RA is
   a. precipitation
   b. hemagglutination
   c. agglutination
   d. hemolysin

10. The IgG bound to latex particles for RF testing is
    a. human
    b. rabbit
    c. horse
    d. a and b

FURTHER ACTIVITIES

Have the students research and discuss RA and its effects on the human body.

Have the students research and discuss SLE and its effects on the human body.

ANSWERS TO REVIEW QUESTIONS

UNIT 1

1. serology
2. c
3. d
4. b
5. a
6. c
7. cd
8. d
9. b
10. a
11. a
12. b
13. b
14. 5
15. a
16. Fc
17. c
18. b
19. c
20. d
21. d
22. d
23. c
24. T cells
25. B cells
26. a
27. a
28. c
29. b
30. a
31. d
32. a
33. b
34. precipitin line
35. c

UNIT 2

1. c
2. a
3. d
4. c
5. a
6. b
7. b
8. c
9. a
10. b
11. d
12. b
13. d
14. b
15. b
16. b
17. c
18. b
19. d
20. d

UNIT 3

1. c
2. a
3. b
4. b
5. d
6. b
7. c
8. a
9. b
10. b
11. d
12. a
13. b
14. c
15. c
16. d
17. c
18. b
19. b

UNIT 4

1. d
2. a
3. d
4. a
5. c
6. a
7. b
8. a
9. a
10. d
11. c
12. b
13. T lymphocytes
14. b
15. Kaposi's sarcoma and mycoplasma pneumonia
16. c
17. a

UNIT 5

1. b
2. a
3. d
4. b
5. d
6. b
7. c
8. a
9. c
10. b
11. c
12. d
13. a
14. b
15. a
16. b
17. c
18. a
19. a
20. d
21. d

UNIT 6

1. b
2. a
3. d
4. a
5. a
6. d
7. c
8. b
9. c
10. d

BIBLIOGRAPHY

Brooks, G.F., et al. *Jawetz, Melnick and Adelberg's Medical Microbiology.* Norwalk, Conn.: Appleton & Lange, 1991.

Bryant, N. J., *Laboratory Immunology and Serology.* Philadelphia: W. B. Saunders Company, 1979.

Davis, N.M., *Medical abbreviations.* Huntingdon Valley, Pa.: Neil M. Davis Associates, 1990.

Henry, J.B., *Clinical Diagnosis and Management by Laboratory Methods.* Philadelphia: W.B. Saunders Company, 1991.

Johnson, A. G., et al. *Microbiology and Immunology.* Baltimore, Md.: Williams & Wilkins, 1989.

Linne, J. J., and Ringsrud, K.M., *Basic Techniques in Clinical Laboratory Science.* St. Louis, Mo.: Mosby, 1991.

Thomas, C. L *Taber's Cyclopedic Medical Dictionary.* Philadelphia: F.A. Davis Company, 1993.

Tilton, R. C., et.al. *Clinical Laboratory Medicine.* St. Louis, Mo.: Mosby, 1992.

Index

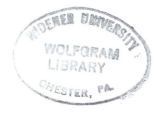